I0380260

Qigong

Find Your Way Towards a More
Effective Yoga

*(Nourshing Exercise Practices for Healing the
Body and Mind)*

Eugene Benedetti

Published By **Eugene Benedetti**

Eugene Benedetti

Qigong: Find Your Way Towards a More Effective Yoga (Nourshing Exercise Practices for Healing the Body and Mind)

ISBN 978-1-77485-447-1

Legal & Disclaimer

The information contained in this book is not designed to replace or take the place of any form of medicine or professional medical advice. The information in this book has been provided for educational and entertainment purposes only.

The information contained in this book has been compiled from sources deemed reliable, and it is accurate to the best of the Author's knowledge; however, the Author cannot guarantee its accuracy and validity and cannot be held liable for any errors or omissions. Changes are periodically made to this book. You must consult your doctor or get professional medical advice before using any of the suggested remedies, techniques, or information in this book.

Upon using the information contained in this book, you agree to hold harmless the Author from and against any damages, costs, and expenses, including any legal fees potentially resulting from the application of any of the information provided by this guide. This disclaimer applies to any damages or injury caused by the use and application, whether directly or indirectly, of any advice or information presented, whether for breach of contract, tort, negligence, personal injury, criminal intent, or under any other cause of action.

You agree to accept all risks of using the information presented inside this book. You need to consult a professional medical practitioner in order to ensure you are both able and healthy enough to participate in this program.

Table Of Contents

Introduction

The health of a person is determined by a variety of aspects. Certain of them are genetic or inheritable. However, many others are influenced by the way we live and the habits we adopt.

It is through them that we are able to become more conscious and develop new practices that help in improving our health and thus our overall wellbeing and quality of life.

Traditional Chinese medicine has its own unique way of assessing the person's health, and determines the various factors which influence the health of a person.

Certain depend on external factors for their needs, like climatic fluctuations as well as the particulars of the region in which we live.

Others are part of our internal like genes, lifestyle (diet and exercise, rest, etc.) and the regulation of our emotions.

For centuries, they believed that the health of an individual could be improved by observing the right habits, which directly impacted the health of a person.

One method they employed to achieve this was through the practice of an exercise routine that later on came as the qigong (pronounced "chi Kung").

The exercises were not just composed of basic movements, but they were also supported by proper respiration and concentration. They were able to keep a healthy blood flow and energetic state which was considered crucial for staying healthy.

In addition, they exercised the mind, body and energy to ensure the total health of the human body.

The basic exercises were constantly developing and, over time, developed into various techniques based on the goal which they were pursuing their participants.

In essence, they kept the energy flow and the working of three aspects as the pillars of their practices.

In the cultivation of three elements (body energy, mind and body) is not limited to the Chinese practice.

Through time, many civilizations have understood the nature of the human being as well as its importance in his activities and his care.

It is relevant that in the tradition of Chinese medicine , it is given an important role and is among its most fundamental concepts.

The various Qigong systems, and, more specifically, those of the Luohan system, are made conscious of the significance of these three elements and devise strategies to improve and enhance them in a balanced and effective method to enhance our wellbeing.

What I'm trying to communicate is the importance of the three components of that we are created and the three ways that can help us enhance them.

In essence, The Three Steps to Health.

What I discuss the contents of this publication is built upon the theories and techniques Luohan Qigong employs for medical treatment.

As I said earlier, it's not only limited to this system, and it can be found in many forms of qigong.

Chapter 1: What Is Qigong?

Qigong (pronounced as Chee-gung) is a Chinese-based practice that originated in China is a potent healing and energy-based system of energy. It is the art and science of gentle movements, meditation and breathing techniques that enhance, cleanse and circulation of Qi (life power). Regular practice of qigong can lead to more energy and better health and a tranquil mental state.

Qigong in the past was referred to as dao yin (guiding energy) or the nei gong (inner work) Qigong's initial name - yang is being revitalized. Yang is a word that means nurturing, and sheng is a word that means life. Yang sheng (qigong) comprises exercises for healing, meditation and methods that promote spiritual, physical, emotional and mental harmony.

Qigong allows practitioners to improve their psychophysiological self-regulation. You are aware of physiological functions that are normally thought to be unnatural, like breathing speed, blood pressure or the circulation of blood and nutrients to organs in the body. Self-regulation allows you to restore your equilibrium, and don't require the aid of a medical device.

Qigong is considered to be one of the most effective ways to improve your health. It only takes about a half-hour to an hour a day to take part in. As a river of immense size, Qigong is supplied by four tributaries: medicine spirituality martial arts, spirituality and the practice of shamanism.

It is possible to understand the reason there isn't an easy definition of such a complicated system of mental and physical development. The practice of qigong as a spiritual one is rooted in the practice of meditation as well as exercise.

Medicine

Chinese medicine includes qigong herbal medicine, acupuncture, diet massage, and diet. Qigong provides self-healing, preventive branch of Chinese medicine. It was and is employed to train practitioners how to be healthier. Hua To (2nd century A.D.) The first guru of Chinese medicine was one of the pioneers of qigong.

Hua To's 'Five-Animal Frolics', which remain popular in the present, follow Tiger, Dear, Monkey, Bear, and Crane's motions. Hua To is associated with a quote about how the body can attain excellent health through gentle exercise and moving every limb.

Spirituality (Buddhism and Taoism)

The Buddhist insists on the importance of diligent practice mindfulness, awareness, and peace are incorporated into the practice of qigong. Many qigong styles were endorsed by Buddhists who needed an exercise and healing method to enhance their long-standing meditation sessions.

Qigong philosophies and practices are outlined in Dao De Jing, the Taoist philosophy classical. Taoists believed that qigong was the best way to achieve their aim of wuji, an unrestricted, alert and inert state of consciousness . It also includes the xing ming shuang that is the practice of keeping the body and the spirit in harmony.

Qigong practitioners as well as Taoists were both looking for a harmony between yin and Yang. Most work in qigong are included in around 1100 Taoist Canon texts.

Martial Arts

Regular qigong training can be beneficial to the sport of martial arts, for instance. Chinese martial artists assisted to develop and improve Qigong techniques as they sought to improve stamina, strength and speed. They also focused on improving the coordination, flexibility and balance and also to strengthen the body to protect itself from injuries.

Shamanism

The book 'The Spring and Autumn Annals' declares that a massive flood - during mythological times - covered a vast part of China and the stagnant waters caused diseases. The Shaman-emperor Yu cleansed the area and divided the waters into rivers by performing the dance of bears and a prayer to the Constellation of Big Dipper's magical power.

As the water drained the people realized that exercising and moving can be akin to the bear dance, causing internal rivers to flow smoothly and clear health obstacles. Qigong practices are discovered on old rock panels across China. Shamans also used these practices and exercises to connect with nature forces and boost divination and healing abilities.

Who is practicing Qigong?

Over 80 million people from China are practicing qigong. There are tens of thousands of practitioners throughout Europe as well as across the United States. Qigong has been thoroughly tested through clinical trials as well as controlled research and is often used as an adjunct to conventional allopathic medical therapies.

Patients with hypertension who do qigong and also take medications have better results than those on medication alone. There is evidence to suggest that qigong can enhance the immune system and mental health and help combating the progression of age-related disabilities. Qigong can be compared to Vitamin C. This enhances the efficiency of enzymes that reduce free radicals (chemicals which cause degeneration of tissues and memory loss).

There are a variety of Qigong styles. Some are designed for general wellness and health, and can be performed daily throughout all of one's life. Qigong also has techniques that are therapeutic and are intended to treat certain ailments.

Qigong is appropriate for both people of all ages, both men and women both young and old active and sedentary and for those who have disabilities. The qigong styles all rest on the same premise of a relaxed and grounded posture with a straight and supple spine, diaphragmatic respiratory (the abdomen retracts upon exhalation and expanding after exhalation) and a calm awareness and fluid movements with little effort.

It is the History of Qigong and Its benefits

Qigong is an integral an integral part of Chinese traditional medicine for centuries. It is a form of qi that functions as the principal aspect of human physiology and psychology, and biology for helping to heal and improve health conditions. Since ancient times, qigong practices throughout China was practiced and proven to work and is available in a variety of forms and styles.

The 3rd century BC book Nan Hua Jing, the philosopher Zhuang Zi explained that the breath of the immortal goes all the way to his feet, while the normal human's breath is restricted to the throat. This is the reason one of the definitions of qigong is breathing.

In China Qigong is an extensive history as a type of traditional exercise used to maintain health and fitness. Certain exercises in qigong like the "Six Healing Sounds" are extremely effective and involve the creation of sounds and their vibrating to cleanse, re-energize and harmonize within the organs of your body. This is how optimal health is achieved.

Qigong also involves meditation. One of the very first Buddhist patriarch Bodhidharma, Da Mo, left India to spread Buddhism during China's Liang Dynasty (from 502 until 557 A.D.). Do Ma is considered as the founder of Buddhism in Chinese

Chan Zong sect ancestor. Then Chan Zong sect was introduced to Japan. Chan Zong sect's training was established in Japan and was later adopted as the country's Zen meditation.

Qigong requires meditation because it is a necessary exercise to help train the mind to control and control the body's energy flow. Once the energy flows it must be coordinated with the mind's actions so that both mind and body are able to benefit from each other's influence and syncronization.

Through mediation, our minds will discern the subtle levels on where the qi is working in the mind and body levels. In recent times For instance, Yan Xin Qigong has been regarded as an qigong practice that is a the form of meditation. Since the past few years, numerous qigong styles that are offered to the public as well as to research purposes are designed to improve general health without mentioning specific connection between particular health conditions and practices.

Qigong's various styles differ in the way they move their bodies, form meditation, breath, and body movement and meditation, but they aren't really practices of internal cultivation centered around qi. Additionally, the various Qigong classes are on textbooks and do not necessarily include the systematic cultivation of qi energy activation, refinement, development, and management.

What is the reason to practice Qigong?

If you are looking for a reliable alternative method to control your health or treat ailments Qigong could be a good option. Qigong has a wealth of advantages. Here are some of the reasons the practice of qigong is effective in modern times.

The cultivation of qi through Tai Chi, which is similar to qigong, is an regular qigong meditation and exercises provide various health benefits

1. Qigong initiates the relaxation response' that is developed by ensuring that the brain is clear of distractions. The relaxation response reduces the autonomic nervous system's activity of the sympathetic nerve, and then dilates blood

capillaries, decreases cardiovascular rate and pressure and improves the flow of oxygen and nutrients to the tissues.

2. Qigong alters the neurochemistry profile towards internal healing that can be accelerated. Also known as information molecules, neurotransmitters bind to receptors within the immune, nervous digestive, endocrine and various other systems to block or stimulate function to increase organ performance, ease pain, reduce cravings for addictive substances and lessen anxiety or depression.

3. Qigong regulates the functions of the pineal, hypothalamus pituitary, and hypothalamus glands, along with the spinal cord and brain's cerebrospinal fluid systems. The cerebrospinal system controls mood and pain , and improves the immune system's function.

4. Qigong introduces theta and alpha (in certain situations) cerebral waves which lower the heart and blood pressure. It helps to improve mental concentration and relaxation. This improves the self-regulating mechanism of the body, by reducing the activity of the sympathetic nervous system.

5. Qigong helps balance the right and left brain hemispheres. It enhances mental clarity, decreased anxiety and a deeper sleep.

6. Qigong boosts the efficiency of tissue regeneration as well as cell metabolism through the increasing the flow of nutrientand oxygen-rich blood to the organs, tissues, and the brain.

7. Qigong increases the immune system's effectiveness by increasing the flow and speed of lymphatic fluid as well as the activation of immune cells. Immunity to illness and infection is enhanced by toxic metabolic byproducts eliminated from interstitial spaces within the glands, organs, and tissues via the lymphatic system.

Chapter 2: 3 Steps To Our Well-Being

In this moment in an overview, we can see our human nature is made up in a fundamental way of three levels or aspects. While in actuality everything is reduced to energy and empty The different frequencies of energy results in it manifesting in three distinct but interconnected ways: mind, body and energy.

In the end If we focus on these three areas, our life will be more enjoyable more healthy and more enjoyable.

Let's see how can do it;

There are three ways to work with the three treasures of life: breathing, movement, and concentration.

To practice to work on the JING in order to work the JING, which is to describe our physical component is to make use of the movement.

To work on QI, or the energy, we'll make use of breath.

To develop SHEN, our brain will be developed by focusing.

As we learned in the last chapter, for optimal health, it is essential to ensure that all three treasures work in a coordinated and unison manner. So, their work methods should also be healthy. In other words when we exercise to make them truly effective, movements must be synchronized by breathing, and focus.

Although there are some exercises which focus on all three aspects, the remaining two will be always present.

As we've seen many Chinese Qigong systems believe that to keep an optimal state of health it is vital to develop the three treasures, and to maintain the proper flow of energy through the body.

These three techniques will enable us to attain it. They are what we call our "Three Steps to Health and Wellness".

The theories behind a variety of theories, we can see it in the form of "regulating your body's functions, controlling breathing and managing your mind".

Yin Yang; The Importance Of Balance

Before looking into more depth the three instruments or the steps for working to discover the 3 treasures it's crucial to be aware of the theory of yin and Yang. Although it is well-known and well-known, it's important to understand its significance and how it applies to our health and wellbeing and the exercises we can do.

Yin(Yin) as well as Yang (Yang) Yang (Yang) is a philosophical term utilized in the past in China. It refers to a view of the world that is the basis from which Nature and its entire functioning are described.

It is possible to categorize all things that happen within it using this theory. Of course, it's applicable to humans. Its anatomy as well as its behavior can be classified in terms of yin or Yang.

It also provides a theoretical framework that is applicable to the practice of various qigong systems and, of course, to the technique that is presented in this book.

Furthermore, understanding what is yin Yang is crucial to our work and help us achieve one goal or the other in our work. In subsequent chapters, we'll be taught the best way to use this understanding to our exercise and the way it impacts the results.

First, let us examine in a fundamental and clear manner what the significance in this concept.

How do you define YIN-YANG?

Imagine the shape of a hill for a second. The one of the sides has the sun. On the other hand it has shade.

When it is sunny,, there is warmth, light and consequently the activity is higher.

On the other side, the shaded area is a cold, dark and consequently there is more silence.

The part that is sunny is called the yin. The

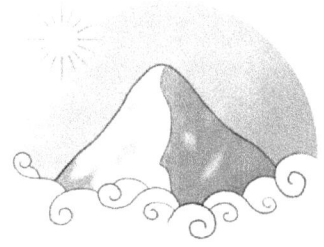

shaded portion can be described as the yin.

As I mentioned earlier the concept of a binary applies to all aspects nature.

In general we can classify everything as yin.

- mobile

Hot!

- rising

- centripetal

- bright

Outward

- low

- Business

We can categorize it as the yin

Motionless

- chilled

- descending

- - centrifugal

- obscure

- In the inland

- deep

- - respite

Human beings cannot get around this rule. The book Su Wen (an ancient Chinese medical text) declares: "any tissue structure of the human body could split into two distinct parts , which are represented by the"yin-yang".

Let's take a look at various examples from this class;

Yang: man, an element of our body. upper portion either exterior or surface energy, entrails etc.

Yin: woman anterior-medial portion of body. portion internal organs, blood, etc.

It is true that this concept can be applied to Qi Gong exercises. Let's take a general look at some examples of how to categorize some moves;

Yang: to stimulate to be energised, to relax, to climb, etc.

Yin means to let your breath out, relax, fall, etc.

However, we should keep at all times that the yin the yang nature of an thing or activity is not absolute, but rather relative. In other words, it is the opposite of yin or Yang in relation to an additional element.

It is also crucial to realize that yin and Yang are not two distinct kinds of energy, but represent two opposing poles however, they are simultaneously, they are they are both complementary to each other.

The interdependence between the two elements can be perfectly illustrated by the famous Taiji sketch (supreme essential):

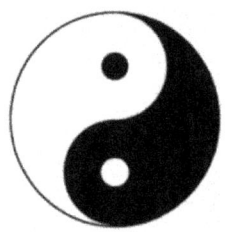

We can observe the principal elements of this interdependence.

Yang and yin are two opposites. Everything has its own opposite however this isn't absolute, but it is relative since there is nothing that is entirely Yang.

- Yin and yang are interdependent. They are not able to exist without one in isolation. For instance we are provided by daytime, but can't exist without night.

Yin and Yang may be subdivided further into yin the other. Each aspect of yin or Yang can be subdivided into Yang for a long time. For instance the sunniest portion of a mountain can be thought to be to be yang. There are some things that can be classified as momo more yin or Yang more.

- Yang and yin are both consumed and generated by one another. The two forms an equilibrium that is dynamic: as one grows and the other is reduced, both decrease. It is not a problem that is unintentional in that when one is growing too much, it causes the other one to concentrate on itself, which in the end time causes a change. For instance, when it is sunrise, sun gets brighter until the darkness disappears completely. Once it has reached its maximum brightness, it starts to dim down until it is dark.

Yin and Yang are able to become opposites. In the case of the previous instance the day gets transformed into night , and night turns into day in a constant cycle. Another instance could be the transition of seasons. The colder seasons are followed by the heat, and the reverse is true.

In yin is yang, and in yang it is the yin. In yin there is always something yang however in yang there's a little bit of the yin. This is symbolized by tiny circles that are different colors.

- Yin and yang are relative. The thing or natural phenomenon can be described as either yin or yang based on what you are comparing it to. For instance water that is fluid state can be Yin to steam, and the opposite is true for the ice.

There are many examples of nature where the principles of conflict, alternation and transformation are apparent;

The dawn is believed to be an ascending in the energy Yang, which attains its peak at noon. From then from then, it begins to fall while the yin energy rises to its highest at midnight. The yin energy begins to diminish and the yang increases and repeats the same process that yin and Yang are controlled and alternate to ensure a equilibrium.

It is not difficult for us to discover more details on the theory of yin and Yang. We have already seen that it applies to all areas of our lives. There are genuine philosophical currents on this theory. However, I believe that the information provided to date is sufficient. I believe it's better to concentrate on how we can apply the theory to our body and also to our qigong practice.

There is one principle I believe is essential to be able to hold on to;

It is possible to practice qigong in a balance as well as in a yin manner as well as in a yin manner.

Balanced form. The exercises are practiced to maintain that balance of yin Yang to achieve a neutral effect.

Yang form; we'll focus more on the phase or Yang aspects of the exercise in the hope of strengthening, toning, or raising the intensity.

The Yin Form We will focus on the yin or phase elements of the practice in the hope of relaxing or sedating the level of energy.

It is a general concept to comprehend how the concept of yin and yang can assist us in reaching our objectives. There are occasions that we must be active and increase our energy. Some times we just want to unwind, release tensions. However there are times when we desire to use on the 3 treasures of life in a harmonious way.

While there are some exercises that are designed to accomplish one goal or another, minor variations in the implementation of these can have a different impact.

In the next section, we will look at how to create a balanced, neutral exercise that has a yang effect or yin impact based on our preferences.

Chapter 3: Beginning Position

There are many times when people are drawn in practices such as Qigong or Taiji (tai chi) in hopes of learning how to relax. However, while this is not the intention of these methods however, it is an actual necessary condition for a successful practice. We'll dive a bit further into this matter in the future.

Being in a good posture is essential for this. Learning to be in a good posture is the very first step in the majority of traditional methods of energy work.

There's even a well-known method in the qigong as well as Taiji systems, called zhan zhuang (literally translate to "standing still as if the stake") that consists of sitting still, inactive to a particular position, in order to improve our posture, removing tensions that are not needed, enhancing flow of Qi calm the mind, and prolonging and long.

This time, we're not going to take on that task. We'll simply determine the initial position from which we can begin all of the exercises.

It is important to be aware of how important it is to maintain balance, the concept of yin and Yang. Extremes can be harmful and an excessive amount of tension could be the same as excessive relaxation. One of the major goals of the postures we will learn is to get ourselves in a position that is as well-balanced as is possible.

Posture for the Feet

We will stand up straight. The feet should be about shoulder width apart. The toes of your feet slightly to the side. The knees were stretched, but were not blocked. The pelvic waist is in neutral position with a slight retroversion to the sacrum. The back straight with a appearance of the front. Arms are relaxed and naturally hang towards the sides, so that the middle fingers are lightly touching the sides of the legs.

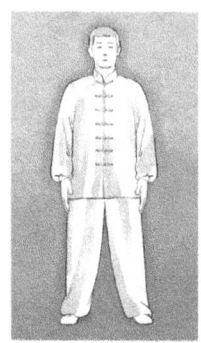

Sitting Position

The posture of sitting is slightly more Yin than standing position. Traditionally , it was done with the legs crossed and sitting on a cushion. However, for the majority of people, it's more comfortable, and generally equally efficient, to sit in the chair.

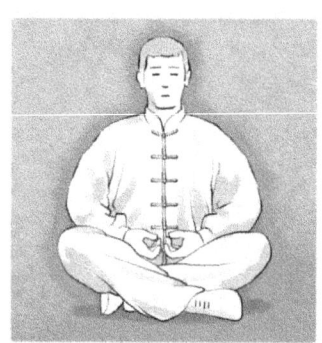

In this scenario it is recommended to be seated at the edges of your chair and avoid leaning against the backrest. The ideal is for the knees to be bent at 90 degrees, so that your knees are in line with the floor. It is also possible to tilt them but always with legs lower that the knees and never the reverse. The feet remain wider than the shoulders with the tips slightly to the side or even completely in line. The back is straight, and we keep our attention towards the front. The arms are naturally relaxed, however the way we position them is an order that the wrists are resting on the legs. As of now, in an ideal position, the hands can be positioned either up or down however, they must be at ease.

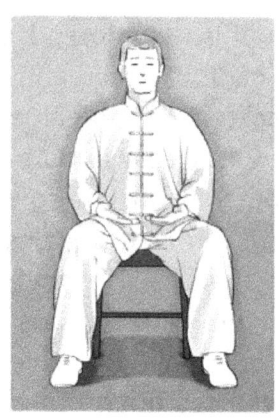

Step 1.-Jing Work

To really enhance our physical condition it is vital to move. Actually, we can take part in any exercise we enjoy and is good for us. Walking, running or dancing or doing any other sport regularly, moderately and most importantly aerobically will help to improve our health and strengthen our jingle.

However, the aim of Qigong is a bit more. There are times when we don't just speak about strengthening as well as regulating or balancing our body. We must be aware that on one hand, we are trying to strengthen our jing however, we also wish to increase the flow of energy throughout our body. Moving is a great instrument to improve blood circulation, and consequently energy all over the body.

Although any exercise will help the circulation of blood however, there are certain methods that are more efficient and suitable for it.

In qigong the body's equilibrium is typically achieved through an assortment that includes stretching exercises and relaxing that allow us to remove tension from the body. This can lead to an ideal state of relaxation.

Relaxation that the body experiences is necessary for a healthy posture to allow blood and energy to flow freely. It also allows us to breathe in a controlled manner and keep a healthy mental state.

This kind of exercise consists of exercises that stretch or relax different body parts in a slow and steady manner to increase circulation.

There are numerous benefits we can reap from the stretching exercises which include this type of. In addition to increasing the energy circulation various tissues or structures within the human body can benefit;

* Muscles;

As the primary part of our locomotor system they are among the structures that benefit from stretching.

Stretching aids in the correct movement of the muscles' structures. the muscles, which in turn ensures their effectiveness.

They aid in maintaining flexibility, adaptability, and elasticity. These factors define the strength of muscles.

They can help prevent contractures, which can improve the overall function of the muscles.

One of the most fascinating results we can get from the stretching exercise is draining. when we compare the muscles as a sponge which is full of blood, every time we stretch it , it helps to drain it, removing the blood within as well as eliminating the waste products. When we relax and release the stretching, just as the sponge would do it, the muscle is filled with blood. This time, it is it is oxygenated and receives more nutrients. This way, we can increase blood flow, and thus energy levels within the various muscle groups, increasing their nutrition as well as the elimination of waste products along with the many benefits this implies.

They aid in achieving a proper balance of reciprocity between agonists and antagonist.

* Joints and bones

Stretching stimulates synovial glands and results in the creation of synovial fluid. This helps the tissues that are being nourished by synovial fluids and joint surfaces in particular.

When we stretch during the majority of exercises, what you want to achieve is to create a separation between the various bones that comprise every joint. In other words expanding the interarticular space in a flash as shown in the diagram. This causes a series of compressions-decompressions that also contribute to a better nutrition of the articular cartilages.

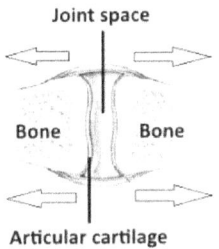

Joint space

Bone   Bone

Articular cartilage

This allows joints to be freed up which aid in the process of regenerating bone. This is particularly important for the spinal column because even when we're not doing anything it helps to reduce that space in between vertebrae.

Additionally the intra-articular temperature gets elevated, which means it is possible that synovial fluid gets less viscous, and can perform its duties better.

It has been proven that moderate physical activity can help in reducing depletion of bone mass.

In favor of more elastic muscles , and avoiding contractures, we are able to remove tensions and pressures from the bones, and thus avoid one of the causes that favor bone wear.

* Ligaments;

The decompression or separation of the ligaments we discussed earlier exposes to tensions that are specific to the various ligaments, whose purpose is specifically, to keep the joint in a united state. The controlled tension to which they are exposed helps strengthen the ligaments.

* Tendons;

Another great benefit of these exercises is the tendon. As I've said before stretching a muscle actively requires contracting its antagonists. Furthermore, following the phase of exercise during which we achieve the highest stretch, we let it relax and then contract until it is at an extent at which we begin another stretch. The result is that stretching commences by contracting the muscle, transforming the muscle in its initial phase in to an eccentric stretch. The stretches, as the muscles are still contracted initially and has a particular impact on the tendon that makes it more flexible and resilient.

In reality, eccentric stretching is a powerful therapeutic tool for massage therapy and physiotherapy in treating tendon disorders.

Tendons are among the least understood structures used in various physical tasks. Qigong practice can help to fill in this gap.

PRACTICE

It can be difficult to show with a manual the correct method of executing the exercises.

The following is a simple yet very effective example of how stretching can improve circulation of Qi in addition to improving our Jing.

It is a very well-known practice and can be found in a variety of variations in the majority of qigong systems.

In the following link (https://youtu.be/oxEzkMD1Oys) you will accede to a video in which you will be able to see its execution. Along with the instructions below, you'll be able to make it simple to master.

For the beginning, take the first starting position that we have ever seen, the one where we are sitting.

It is a good idea to examine your posture, and see if you are in accordance with the instructions given in the chapter that corresponds to it. In the future, after we've talked about it, you'll be able spend just a few minutes controlling your breathing as well as your mind. At present, it's sufficient to concentrate on your posture, and be attentive to the sensations you're experiencing.

In this position, while keeping your arms in a relaxed position, connect your fingers and then place them on your stomach, with your palms in a downward direction. While doing this you should bend your knees slightly. Maintain your back straight, and straight ahead. (fig. 1).

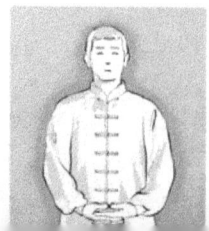

Figure 1.

Begin stretching your legs, and at the same time, raise your palms up in front of you until your forearms touch the ground. (fig.2)

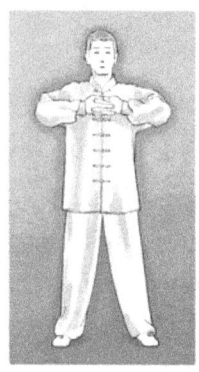

Figure 2.

From this point on you can continue raising your hands and turn your palms until your hands are looking upwards.

Continue to work upwards to the point that your arms are completely stretched. You've stretched your legs out, your back straight, your arms stretched to the max with your hands just above your head , and your palms up (fig.3).

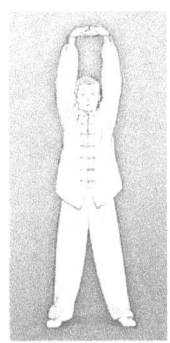

Figure 3

Maintain this position for a few seconds while allowing the intention (Yi) to push upwards, regardless of whether there isn't any further movement since it has at its maximum extension.

In the end, only if you are able to maintain your balance, walk on tiptoes in the direction to reach a little higher. Be sure to not only move with the hands but your thoughts, using your goal. (fig. 4)

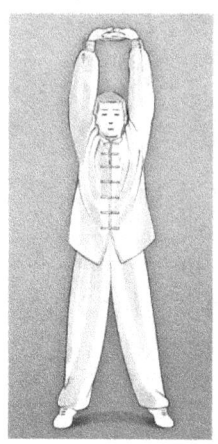

Figure 4.

Once you have done this, place your feet down on the floor, let go of your hands and slowly move your arms to the side until you get to the bottom, then return to the original position (Fig. 5, 6). Your knees should be bent slightly while they lower the weight of your arms. Your mind's concentration also becomes relaxed, with your attention now on the sensations relaxation brings when you stretch.

We can repeat this our mantra as many times as we'd like.

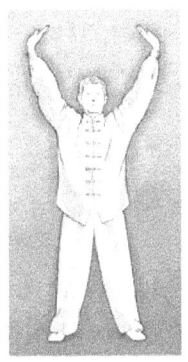

Figure 5

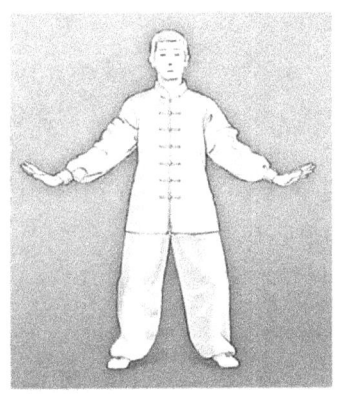

Figure 6

The purpose of this exercise is to stretch the entire musculature the trunk. This, as we've previously seen it will result in the increased flow of nutrients and blood.

But we also subject the internal organs to a kind of pressure-decompression, producing a pumping effect, which will also benefit from a better blood supply and energy.

The most important aspect is the stretching of the spinal column that aims to relax for a short time the vertebrae and thus help to improve the condition of the various structures they rely on (discs and ligaments.).

Additionally, we stretch the muscles in the arms and legs.

This practice allows us to be more alert, but simultaneously, we feel more at ease. It is best at first to not be thinking about your breathing however we'll see how your body naturally breathes when you bend your arms. It also lets out air when you stretch and relax your arms.

Keep your eyes on the your direction during the workout. It helps to stay standing straight and remain in balance while walking. Be patient and don't rush to perform the move and be mindful of the sensations created. Be aware of how important it is to maintain balance and avoiding excessive tension while stretching and a lot of relaxation while releasing.

Repeat the exercise several times, and you'll discover that you have a way of remembering the cycles of the seasons or days and you will be able to follow the concept of yin and Yang. Beginning with the relaxation at the start of the movement (yin) it starts to increase and expand until it reaches its maximum extension (yang) then from there , it shrinks until it reaches its lowest point to begin the cycle.

Step 2.-Qi Work

For the work specific to the qi element it is necessary to make use of breathing. While, as we see, the movement and concentration are also helpful in mobilizing energy to go wherever we wish within our system, the role of various types of breathing to complete this goal is particularly important.

According to the traditional Chinese medical practices, breathing triggers the movement of qi within the body. Through breathing, we are in a position to increase or slow down the rate of our heart (by breathing in short or long breaths). This is why we recognize that breathing can alter the flow of blood, and consequently the flow of energy.

To improve our breathing, we need to be aware of it and manage it. The way we breathe is constantly affected by various factors like conversation or emotional issues, bad postures, fatigue and stress, making it often excessively superficial.

Since breathing is the primary source of boosting energylevels, unsteady, distracted, and shallow way of breathing can negatively impact the vitality of our bodies.

So, to regulate and allow the flow of energy (and together with it the blood, with all of its nutrients) throughout our body, it is vital to be in control and regulate breathing.

Let's take a look at some of the main benefits that breathing exercises provide us with;

According to the theories of traditional Chinese medicine it is believed that breathing is the primary driver of the qi. This is why the improvement of our breathing can help to increase the flow of energy and, because of it, blood flow throughout our body.

They result in an increase in the lung's elasticity, and thus their breathing capacity. This effect is sustained throughout the day, not just during the exercise of exercises.

It boosts the oxygenation levels of the entire body as well as the tissues within it, which contributes in this manner to enhance the performance of the various systems. This leads to a better flow of the tissues and to eliminate waste.

By the movements of various muscles we utilize to breathe, particularly the diaphragm, our internal organs get a massage. This stimulates blood flow through the organs (kidneys and livers, spleens the heart, kidneys ...).

Exercises in breathing can assist us achieve more tranquility and peace of mind. Yet, you can also help to achieve an increase in focus as well as mental clarity.

Breathing exercises do not just assist us in bringing energy to various locations or points however, we also get various effects from it like the speed of or the rate at which the flow of blood.

Thus, there are many different breathing styles in qigong, that we'll use based on the outcome we would like to attain.

Two Fundamental Ways To Breathe

One of the primary goals that we will be pursuing it is to assist us channel the energy towards various areas.

There are two kinds of breathing that can aid us in mobilizing your energy to a specific manner. In other words that they will alter the motion of the Qi and the areas in which we intend to control it.

Let's look at these two kinds of breathing are.

A) Linear or natural breathing

B) Breathing at heights or zones

A. Natural Or Linear Breathing

In this form of breathing, it is simple to breathe through the nose and exhale out of the mouth. This is why we refer to it as natural breathing. We also refer to it as linear breathing due to the result we experience at the energy level. the moment we breathe,, energy is increased and when we breathe out, energy decreases in a linear fashion.

It is the most basic form of breathing that we can start to begin to work.

First, it is important to train the practitioner to be aware of his or her breathing. At first, without movement, and then through the various exercises, we will be able to recognize the rhythm of our breathing. As we progress, we'll attempt to make our breathing deeper , but not without pushing it.

This is where we begin to practice what I refer to as"the "concept of the bottle" by imagining the body (actually your lungs) are as a bottle which is about to be filled. If we put the bottle in the tap it'll fill up from bottom and, when we turn it for emptying, this will happen to the top that is first empty. If we are filling our lungs up with air (which is reflected by the movement in our body) the lungs will start to fill from the bottom upwards as we exhale. When we do this in the same manner as this bottle shows, it will be the bottom part will be first to be empty.

When we are able to breathe deeply, with pauses, relaxed and in the way that we just witnessed then we can begin to include different forms of breathing. This includes, for instance breathing yang as well as yin type and so on. In the future, I will explore the various breathing techniques.

B. Breathing for Heights or Zones

The most commonly used method is to breathe naturally and unconsciously, with no attention paid to the process.

We can also take control, and soon we'll recognize that in order to breathe, is dependent on the action of several muscles.

Based on the muscles we utilize, the air will be directed towards different parts of our lung, causing different impacts on our bodies. In many Qigong systems three breathing styles are generally distinguished according to the musculature we utilize and the part of the lungs to which the air is directed.

The LOW ZONE is usually called diaphragmatic breath or abdominal. It is controlled by the diaphragm's movements. When it is stimulated, it moves downwards, bringing the air into the most deep part of the lung. The abdominal organs to move outward and down upon inspiration, then return to their original position upon expiration. This causes a process of massage or pumping. through this we get a more efficient circulation of blood, and consequently energy in the lower region in our bodies. By using the terminology from Chinese medical practices, one could describe it as activating on the lower Jiao. This will strengthen all the tissues within this area, particularly the internal organs involved.

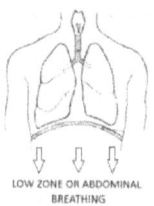

LOW ZONE OR ABDOMINAL
BREATHING

* MEDIUM ZONEis is also known as thoracic, (or intercostal) breathing. It relies on intercostal muscles that sit within the middle of the ribs. In the course of inspiration, these muscles grow and push the ribs forward and widening the ribs. In exhalation, the muscles return back to their normal state. In this way, we aid in ensuring that to circulate energy and blood through the middle part of our body. This is in Chinese medicine is called Jiao Medium. In turn, all tissues in this zone are benefited by it, and in particular those organs inside it.

MIDDLE ZONE OR THORACIC
BREATHING

* HIGH ZONE Sometimes called clavicular respiratory. It is the clavicles that breathe in a rising direction, expand the upper part of the lungs and allow the air to to the zone. After exhalation, they relax, and then return to their

normal position. Thus, it is the entire upper region as well as the organs within the body, that benefit from the massage or pumping that is produced through breathing. According to Chinese medicine, we'll refer to it as treating on the upper Jiao

HIGH ZONE OR CLAVICULAR
BREATHING

In essence, is our goal is to get air to all of the heights we've observed. This is how the muscles that are responsible for controlling the flow of air to each of them are contracted and relaxed and create tension and relaxation of the organic structures found at each of the higher peaks.

It creates an effect like the one you get with massages; it will increase the circulation of blood and energy that is distributed to the high points. This improves the performance and health of the entire region and the associated internal organs. This is due to increased blood supply, which will result in greater nutrition for the tissues in general and improve removal of waste.

Six Breathing Systems

As we've just witnessed the two fundamental breathing methods help control the flow of Qi and the regions where we wish to work.

With the breath, we can have various effects on the energy, independent of the area where we are in.

Even though we're not conscious, the breathing cycle is made up in four phases distinct from each other: Inspiration exhalation, pause and pause.

By altering the duration and/or intensity of each one of them, we can create different effects on our bodies.

In the traditional Luohan qigong , the six breathing methods or techniques are taught in conjunction with the corresponding goals.

Let's look at which of the six breathing systems.

1. Breathing that is balanced (neutral)

2. Yang type breath

3. A type of breathing called Yin

4. Exhalation breathing (pao sik)

5. The Turtle Breathing (quai sik)

6. The Embryonic Breathing (reverse)

But FIRST...BREATHE through the nose or Through THE MOUTH?

Again, it all depends on the goal we hope to accomplish. The nose is designed specifically to breath, and it is responsible to filter and heat the air.

The mouth allows us to take more air into and out.

As a rule of thumb generally speaking, you breathe out and in through your nose whenever you wish to keep the energy within more, and also when you notice that the Qi motion you're looking for is not as strong.

It is also recommended to do this to do this when it is extremely cold and we have to get the air heated. From the perspective of energy the act of inhaling and exhaling with the nose have an invigorating effect on the Qi.

If we breathe through the nose, and exhale through our mouths We tend to have more qi movement since the air will be released more easily through the mouth. As a rule of thumb when we breathe this way when we breathe through the nose, we raise the qi. When exhaling through our mouths, we reduce the Qi.

It is also possible to inspire with the mouth. While it's not the best option in everyday life, there are instances when we could utilize it. Particularly, when we require larger intake of air. In situations, like the case of exertion, the body is able to take in air from the mouth in a natural manner since it permits greater intake of this, and consequently a greater flow of oxygen.

In more advanced forms of Luohan Qigong, one breathes with one's mouth in order to guide the air into concrete zones or areas.

It is interesting to observe that there are equipment for the rehabilitation of patients suffering from diverse ailments. Patients need to blow in the direction to move a number of balls inside. The device is utilized to improve lung capacity and strength and, in these exercises, is inhaled and exhaled using the mouth. This enables us to realize that even though it's not the best way to breathe from day day however, in certain situations it is totally acceptable using the breath through the mouth.

Let's take a examine the six kinds of breathing.

Breathing Balanced

Beginning with the reality that we know the concepts about Yin and Yang and Yang, we can describe balanced breathing as one which has a neutral influence on our body.

This means that this is not a way to seek to activate our bodies (yang) and also relax ourselves (yin) The thing we're looking for is an equilibrium or neutral impact. We want to increase the flow of energy however, in a balanced manner.

In order to achieve this, we'll concentrate on the power of our inspiration that lasts exactly like the exhalation. For general basis, we'll count to three each time we breathe in, and we can also do the same each time we exhale. Naturally, this three-digit count will vary in speed or duration dependent on the individual's lung capacity. It's just an issue of counting to ensure that inspiration and exhalation remain the same.

A balanced breathing practice is a fundamental technique that can help us to relax, concentrate and become more aware of our body, as well as relieve tension and improve flow of qi.

Remember that you shouldn't hold your breath for long periods of time. In general, it is recommended not to fill your lung with more than 70% from their maximum capacity. This can prevent unnecessary tensions and use more of the air we breathe.

Take a moment to feel an inspiration by filling up all your lungs. Soon you will notice that you're strained and are forced to let the air out quickly without control over the exhalation.

The goal is to become aware of breath, and to learn how to control it. We also "play" using the 4 phases of it to get different results.

Instead of filling the lung completely, we fill about 70 percent of it and we be able to hold the air for longer if we'd like and can then regulate the expiration better and alter it to be longer and shorter, more intense or soft as per our desires.

Practice

Take either of these two possible starting positions that we have observed. You can stand or sit, depending on which is the most comfortable for you.

Take a few moments or as long you think is necessary to concentrate on your body, and analyzing the areas we noticed that are shoulder-width apart; feet with your back straight with arms relaxed, and looking towards the future. Keep your eyes open, but I suggest that you close them slightly to help keep yourself away from distractions and concentrate on you.

After you have stabilized your body, you can concentrate on breathing. In the moment take a deep breath through your nose, and exhale through your nostrils or your nostrils, whichever is the most comfortable for you. Take note of your breath and be aware of the four phases, which are occurring in a cyclical manner. Slowly, increase your breathing longer, deeper as well as more relaxed and regular, while avoiding filling your lungs to the max and making sure the way you breathe out you don't blow your entire breath out.

Do not be concerned if initially you are distracted or your thoughts wander elsewhere. If you are aware of it just focus on breathing.

After a time it can take several minutes, or after the practice of a few breaths We will be aware of the length that our breaths take. We can try to make both the inhalation and the inspiration be the same. For a reference, you can count up to three times as you breathe in, and up to three each time you exhale.

This will result in an even effect on the Qi. We just have to make the qi circulate (in addition to the benefits we have seen breathing exercises can bring) However, in a way that is more neutral.

Yang Breathing

When we breathe this way, we can make the inhalation longer than exhalation. Similar effects could be accomplished by putting greater emphasis on inspiration (making it more powerful).

To accomplish our aim, we should count up to four times when we inhale and 3 when we exhale.

The effect we receive from this breathing technique is a yang-related effect; increasing energy, stretching the body, increasing circulation, etc.

Practice

Like the previous exercise select the starting point that feels most comfortable to you. Take a few minutes to concentrate and control your breathing. After a few times be aware of the time and allow the inspiration to be slightly longer in comparison to the exhalation. As mentioned, a great method is to count four during the inspiration phase and three or more for the exhalation.

Through it, we'll get an increase in toning as well as more yin. It can help us be more active, increase our energylevels, and to rejuvenate our bodies, etc.

Breathing Yin

When we breathe this way, it is possible to get an opposite effect. We achieve a yin-like effect and lower the energy level as well as relax the body and calm the circulation, etc..

In order to accomplish this we'll make the inspiration shorter and the exhalation shorter. This time it could also be worthwhile to place more focus in exhalation (making it more powerful or prominent).

In the meantime, counting beads will be done. We'll use a number of three them to three while breathing in, and four when we breathe out.

Practice

The exact same way as the previous versions, however, after taking a regular, starting posture and paying close attention to breathing, we'll focus on the time, and count from three to four when we inhale as well as up to 4 times when exhaling.

This provides us with the ability to relax, soothe and sedative effects. Also, it creates an increased yin effect.

Just by doing this kind of breathing that is basic and knowing the concept of yin and Yang, we've already observed how we can create various effects on our bodies by making minor changes in the duration of different breathing phases.

It's something fundamental easy, yet helpful in our training. What we've seen can be used for any exercise when we understand it properly is the best way to adapt it to our needs according to the type of work we want to do in a more vigorous or stimulating way, or to work more relaxed and softer way or just want to perform a more balanced work.

In times when we require more energy (tiredness or apathy.), practicing yang type breathing can help us.

In contrast to situations in which we have to unwind (stress anxiety, tension anxiety, stress, etc.) breathing in a yin-like manner can be beneficial.

If we just want to increase energy levels, concentrate your mind, and enhance overall health and wellbeing the practice of breathing in a balanced way is sufficient.

Another method is to change our breathing that is neutral into yin or yang:

A faster breathing rate will cause us to perform an easier breathing which can result in a yin effect, which will help to increase our heart rate, our energy levels, etc. Contrarily the slower breath will result in us breathing more deep, which can result in an increased Yin effect as well as more relaxation, decrease the heart rate, etc..

Quai Sik (Turtle Breathing)

As we've seen that the respiratory system is comprised of four phases.

Inspiration-pause-expiration-pause

In the past, we've observed how we can alter the time of inspiration and expiration based on our requirements.

We can also make use of the existing pauses between two periods to reach certain goals.

The known as "quai sik" or breathing technique of turtles consists of holding breath. In other words, we lengthen the length of certain breaks to meet a certain purpose.

In a broad sense we could claim that in the Luohan Qigong practice, we utilize this breathing method in order to keep the energy or qi within an area for the specified duration. The amount of time that we retain we use in our practice generally is quite short typically just a couple of seconds. It's typically done with a break during the exercise we're doing , and then focusing on the location or area that we wish to hold the focus.

There are two variations of this kind of breathing and the other is when we take a pause following inspiration, and the other one that we perform after exhaling. Let's look at a bit more in depth each of the two.

1. It is about invigorating, holding the air, and then release it. It produces a more yin effect, which means that we try to tone the area or point we're working on.

2. This time we exhale, and then we stop and then continue in a state of inspiration. In this case, it's an yin-like effect. It is our goal to hold the qi in a certain region or point, however with a more relaxed intention.

Practice

Start by establishing a new position. Spend a few minutes to be aware of your breathing.

When you are at a point where you feel comfortable to be inspired, hold it for just a few minutes. In the beginning just one or two seconds should be sufficient. Do not exceed three seconds. Don't make retentions longer without supervision from an experienced professional.

There are numerous benefits that this little retention offers us. At the energy level in Qigong, it is an invigorating, accumulator Qi. A teacher of mine would claim that he was using it to "build the qi".

After that, take some balanced breaths. After a few times then take a brief breath following expiration. They follow the same guidelines that they did before. The duration of between three to five minutes is enough. It will be evident that the result you experience this time is more relaxing and more Yin.

Pao Sik (Breathing With Explosion)

This breathing method involves releasing air quickly following an inspiration. It is generally employed for the purpose of relaxing tension and encouraging the circulation of Qi. It helps to relax and facilitates the removal of blocks to the blood circulation and energetic flow.

This can be very beneficial when you are dealing with anxiety or stress, stiffness, mental and physical tension.

It is often used in conjunction along with the technique of quai sik, or turtle breathing. Also, after an inspiration, we'd keep our breath for a couple of seconds before suddenly releasing the air.

By combining this technique, we can to channel the energy into one specific area, to achieve a relaxing effect , and ensure that the energy to circulate in a proper manner. It is possible to strengthen the qi at same time we are able to relax the muscles.

We have two methods to perform this kind of breathing.

The first method is eliminating all the air has been a source of inspiration previously. By doing this, we experience an increased feeling of being clearing the blockage, however it comes with the disadvantage that when repeated, it causes a significant loss of Qi.

The other way to do it is to exhale only a small amount of air immediately after inspiration and then follow with an exhalation that is normal, less tense and controlled.

The most commonly used version of both, because it lets you relax an area, without losing the qi.

Practice

Pick a posture to start from. It is important to take some time to concentrate and control your breathing. It is now time to breathe through your nose and exhale out of your mouth. After a few times then breathe in, create the air retain for a short time, then let go of a portion of the blow. Continue exhaling the air that you've got. The sound may be heard when you release a portion of the air using an exhalation. It is normal.

You'll notice a rejuvenating impact as and a restful one. It helps to ease tension.

Breathing in Embryonics (Reverse)

Reverse breathing refers to something that, in contrast to normal breathing that when we breathe in the abdomen, we contract it by pushing all the abdominal walls towards the inside. When we exhale, these walls stretch outwards towards the outside, like we were relaxed.

This causes more pressure on internal organs as to the pressure that is exerted by the diaphragm upwards when breathing, we add on the pressure that is exerted by the abdominal walls to the side. This allows us to enhance the pumping and massage effect the muscles exert on all the internal organs while breathing.

In our system , it is also referred to as embryonic breathing since we tend to put our mind or attention on the navel when it comes to realisation. This way, we can focus our efforts specifically on the Jing (essence).

Practice

Start by laying down. Then, join your palms and then place them on top of your navel. Do a few slow and relaxed breaths. You'll notice that breathing in increases the abdomen, while breathing out expands the abdomen.

You can reverse this process. breathe in but don't let your abdomen expand. Instead, deliberately push it towards the back. After you have let out the air, ease it out and let it expand. It may initially be a bit strange and may even cost you, but with time, it will begin to come out more effortlessly.

Personally, I love doing this kind of exhalation using the nose, both when I breathe as well as when exhaling.

There will be a stronger abdominal contraction when you breathe in and also a stronger release as you let out the air. This will allow you to compress the qi further, i.e. draw it closer to your lower abdominal region. Also, it can increase the pressure on the organs of the abdomen.

We've already looked at the two types of breathing and the six ways of breathing.

You can employ any of these six techniques to the two breathing forms that we have seen in breathing.

This means that we can create an organic or linear breath, linear type neutral, or the yin kind. Additionally, we can include pao sik, quai sik, and create embryonic.

The same can be done with the different heights.

The possibilities are endless However, when we practice and get used to it, we'll be able to see the possibilities of combinations that are more sensible and will typically appear in the various Qigong exercises.

Step 3.-Shen Work

As we have seen earlier shen can be a broad concept that is far over what Westerners think of as "mind". When we talk about shen, in addition to the actual mental activity we also talk about the various manifestations of the person's vitality. the way they look, their manner of speaking, etc.

To accomplish the task of our shen, we'll make use of concentration. In addition, we will be working on the Chinese concept known as "YI" meaning "intention".

In ancient qigong concepts it is commonly believed"that "wherever you are in your head where the mind is, there the qi will be". This is the basic and most crucial concept of shen training.

Thus, our goal should be to master the art of directing our minds to places in which we wish to channel our energy.

We also recognize that the things we think about grows. Also you attract what you think about. So, a calm, positive and focused mindset about what we're doing will help effectively circulate the qi.

The thing we're trying to accomplish with the majority of Qigong practices is paying complete attention to what we do. Our intention or mind, i.e. our YI, should be connected to breathing and movement constantly.

A focus on the presentmoment, and on what we're doing each and every moment, while in harmony with breathing and movement will assist us in having an improved hern (mind).

In certain Eastern beliefs, the mind is often compared to an active and playful monkey. The monkey is always on the move and causing trouble. It is impossible to make it remain still as it would be against its natural instincts. We can however give it toys in order to let him be entertained and forget the mischiefs. In this way our brain (monkey) is constantly filled with thoughts and ideas (mischief). We can't eliminate it from thoughts however, we can force it to concentrate on something tangible (toy) in order that it can forget about other thoughts. For instance, focusing for an extended period of time on our breathing could help us be able to forget about other thoughts, since we'd be able to be able to keep it "entretenida".

In some way, it's about controlling where our thoughts want to travel. In our situation, the mind, or more precisely our intentions, should be in sync with our movements and our breathing to help bring Qi to the location of our body that we are working on.

In this manner we can continue to follow the notion that three precious stones shen, jing and qi must be always coordinated.

Practice

As you've observed the work of our minds or, more specifically, of our intentions, or YI, is there constantly. It is present in every action we take. However, let's take a look at an example of how to utilize our minds to guide the qi in certain areas.

In this case, we'll need to choose a starting position. While both we've seen is worth it I suggest you select the sitting posture. It is not necessary to be sitting on a couch by crossing your legs. The correct posture on an appropriate chair is enough.

The goal is to apply the qi principle to three regions which within Chinese medicine are considered to be very significant and can be seen in the photo. There is no need to be familiar with the significance of these areas. For your information I'll explain briefly the purpose behind this;

The three dantians are three areas located in the anterior region of the body. They extend a small distance to the interior. They are not distinct locations, but are slightly bigger zones. It is the Chinese concept of Dantian "(Dan Tian)" comprises two parts:

(Dan) is the presence of a specific substance or elixir that was thought to offer longevity and health.

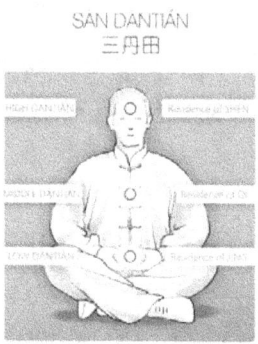

SAN DANTIÁN
三丹田

Let's begin with the first We already have the right posture and have managed our breathing.

In the meantime, prior to launching an idea then we put our mind or our intent into the superior Dantian. It's as if, our minds inform the qi of where we would like it to move. Then we keep on invigorating and keep our focus in the region. After a short breath, we exhale and calm our minds while the air rises. Repeat the procedure 3 or 4 times in each zone and in all three Dantian.

This is just one instance of how we can use intention to direct the flow of qi. It could be useful for any area or point within the human body. Anywhere we pay attention the qi will move.

It is important to recognize that your mind has to be in sync with movement and breathing.

If we are stretching, we should keep our focus on the goal, which will increase the feeling of stretching.

While breathing, the mind can also be a part of and focus on the phases.

Chapter 4: History And How It Functions

The history of Qigong

In the early days one of the terms that were used to define what we now refer to as Qigong used to mean "Tu Na" which translates to "inhalation". The well-known philosopher Zhuang Zi, " in his work Nan Hua Jing (3rd century BC.) clarify that "the immortal's breath is ascended to their feet and the normal person's inhalation is to into the stomach." In the present one of the most commonly recognized terms used to describe Qigong is an exercise in inhalation.

Qigong has a long history throughout China as a regular exercise that helps maintain the health and strength. The Qigong aerobics, known in"the "Six healing Sounds" are a remarkable standard Qigong practice that involves the use of sound and their emotions to cleanse the body, recover, balance and align the organs of the body and thereby achieving optimal health. One of the most significant developments in the history of Qi Gong occurred during the Han Dynasty (200 BC to 500 AD). The reasons for this are the majority of what we think to be the current Qi Gong preparation seems to begin during this time.

In the same time period, Indian Buddhism also set the way for its journey to China in which many of its fundamental beliefs were fused with Taoist beliefs and theories. Additionally, many of the works out techniques were combined and these practices found their way into the call the standard Shaolin Temple practice. In the booming martial arts scene in that time, the art of developing Qi power gained recognition and researched. In actual fact, it is well beyond in the Han Dynasty that the union between Shaolin fitness along with Qi Gong preparation would be working side-by-side. In the Liang Dynasty (500 AD to 1911 AD) connects the modern method in Qi Gong preparation that stimulated perfectly through the 20th century. It would it was then a kind of wellness cultivations which connect modern society with the earlier time of Qigong study.

Deliberation is also a crucial element the Qigong practice. DA MO, the first Buddhist Patriarch Bodhidharma was a native of India to preach Buddhism in China throughout the Liang dynasty (502-557 A.D.). He is regarded as the founder to the Chinese Chan Zong faction of Buddhism. Then Chan Zong was a Chan Zong faction of Buddhism and its method of preparation was introduced to Japan and was later transformed into Zen thinking in Japan. Meditation is an essential practice during Qigong preparation since it is a crucial process for educating the mind to be stay in a straight line and to regulate the flow of energy within the body. When the Qi is activated, it has to be coordinated with the mental behavior so that the intellect as well as the body are able to benefit from the synergy and effects of joint. When the mind is trained through meditation, can detect the subtle levels on where the Qi is working at both the level of the mind and also at that of our bodies. In contemporary times, Yan Xin Qigong is acknowledged as an outline for meditation that is based on Qigong practice.

The undiscovered origins for Qi Gong's origins Qi Gong teaching might, in reality, have several different beginning locations. Some have suggested that the earliest types that comprise Qi Gong aerobics can from Agrarian farmers who were in their understanding of nature. Some have suggested that the origins of aerobics may be from a traditional ritual dance.

Different theories of Qigong

The term "Qigong" is a broad term that covers a range of different methods of exercising. It is actually "energy advancement" which is also known as "energy development". The principal goal of many Qigong techniques is to boost the energy levels of your body and to increase your energy or chi, more evenly and aggregating your capacity to channel it through your plan or use it to perform specific tasks for example, such as contemplation or martial arts. If you join various qigong circles and you'll find different approaches to help you understand the energy of your body that are behind each. Certain circles focus on"the "five elements" an idea that is applied to events that occur in stages, such as the seasons changing. Some circles also employ the acupuncture Zenith model of the body. They are designed to stimulate these lines by a gentle contact or rubbing, slapping non-body-motivation or even images. Some focus on stimulating the different muscles of the body by actions, both small and big and as attention is directed to the human body, the energy begins to flow in certain arrangements.

Three fundamental terms (Jing, Qi, Shen)

Before you can begin any Qigong-related practice it is important to first understand the real meaning of the three treasures: inner energy (jing) and internal energy (qi) and power

73

(shen). They are also known as the three sources or the three lines as they are regarded as the source and origin of your existence.

Jing refers to the spirit, the most distinctive and sophisticated element of everything. Jing is everywhere. It is a symbol of the essential aspect of everything that demonstrates its distinctiveness. Jing is the source of new energy of all living things, and is the one who determines the environment and the traits of that thing. It is the reason for the existence of life.

Qi is the energy that flows through the body. that runs through the human body. Qi is also derived from the exchange of jing you've received from your family members or from the food you consume and the air you breathe.

Shen is the center of your brain. It is the strength of your character. It is the reason you are human because animals don't have a shen. The shen within your body needs to get support from your Qi or energy. If your Qi is strong and complete and your shen is vibrant, it will lighten up.

What is QiGong's effect?

Qigong is the art of refining and manipulating the energy. Through calming the body, it allows the channels to draw in and enhance Qi flow. Additionally, through increasing in compassion, we are able to detect the source of latent disease before it becomes apparent on the physical plane. When we learn to communicate the Qi throughout examination (Yi) we can be taught to help the Qi flow exactly where it's required, and thus prevent the issue before it manifests itself within the body. It is also possible to treat the problem once it is manifested by addressing the cause of the issue (the Qi stagnation or deficiency) through actions that aid in repairing the damage by supplying more Qi and helping to facilitate its flow.

In the event of an injury that is complicated healing, and the tissue fibers have healed in sporadic patterns that make it more likely to be injured again which is a problem that will continue to plague you The slow movements of the beneficial Qigong aligns the injured tissues fibers to the stronger ones, thereby making it stronger. This process is time-consuming.

The body regenerates itself on a regular basis. This is the reason why Qigong is a successful exercise should be practiced each throughout the day, for at least one hundred days. Within a time of a hundred days, new relationships have been established within the brain (called neuropeptides) and a change in the chemical system takes place in the body that permits Qigong to flow along the new way and strengthen itself and develop. This is why healing can be achieved through Qigong. The more severe the wound or condition, the more lengthy the healing process is due to it utilizes the body's natural ability to heal itself.

Chapter 5: The Benefits Of Qigong

Qigong is an Chinese fitness routine built on light movements, meditation and inhalation, offers many benefits, which include improving balance as well as lowering blood pressure. It is alleviating sadness.

Qigong helps strengthen muscles.

Qigong helps strengthen the body quite differently unlike the standard training methods used by Westerners. The aerobics, as well as the energetic stretching build the muscle in a position to stretch and increase flexibility. Qigong, as well as new inner exercises create natural power and flexibility. The sensation of power or feeling "pumped up" you experience during a Western exercise is in reality due to the brawny contracting which blocks the flow of chi. However, the exercise could give you with the utmost flexibility for doing leg splits.

Balance and strengthen all internal organs

Qigong helps build a stronger body, and also to align the internal organs. The majority of people are born with an issue in one or the other organ and qigong has helped correct every move to deal with any individual's specific issue.

Nervous system

The ability of Qigong to build up your nervous system is what makes it an extremely effective method for reducing stress that is present on a daily basis, and also for improving the bodies that haven't been functioning due to prolonged stress.

Normalizing blood pressure

Qigong increases transmission by increasing the suppleness of blood vessels themselves. It is typical in China to advise qigong-based movements to lower and high blood pressure, since both can be caused by problems in vascular stretch and strength.

It is effective for patients with cancer

However, Qigong offers a variety of methods designed for weak people and is, in fact an approach to improves bodily capabilities without movements. Qigong can also be arranged to help cancer patients with a terminal illness as a last option. If they don't have the ability to practice in a sitting or standing position or lying down, they can practice sitting down for a while until energy increases.

Rapid healing

Damage from accidents can occur in a variety of ways, and joints and ligaments are particularly susceptible. Qigong is a gentle stretch and acupuncture-based action, which enhances blood flow as well as energy in the body , which can reduce the impact of injuries and speed up healing. Qigong assists the entire mental and body to relax and relax. Making a practical decision to speed up recovery can decrease the anxiety and irritation.

Control of the physiology

This implies that various areas of the body which were not provoked or in control begin to normalize. For instance inhalation rate and blood heaviness, the rate of breathing hormone levels, and the state of constant discomfort or exhaustion.

Creativity and perception

Perception and creativity produce both and emerge from the same source: an awakened mind and animal, an ability to think in a stomach, to feel with the mind.

Spiritual influences

Qigong's progress is often associated with a range of religious experiences. For instance, synchronicityand significant coincidences, is becoming more frequent. If the Qi is plentiful, clear and smooth, mental sanity is pervaded by sweetness.

No side effects

The effects of healing Qigong aren't as quick as when you take pharmaceutical drugs However, then again, there aren't any side negative effects. The pharmaceutical drugs cause chemical shift, they often trigger an imbalance in the chemical system that causes negative side effects as well as health issues elsewhere within the body, Qigong is often only treating the underlying issue without addressing the root of the problem, which causes it to persist. The issue is that in our modern society individuals want fast results , and do not give their body enough time to recover.

Chapter 6: Qigong Simple Breathing Technique

To Ease Stress

Being able to breathe properly is vital to your overall health. There is no other exercise capable of generating such dramatic and life-changing results, in the amount of effort that is required. It's the deliberate practice of breathing using your whole body in a relaxed or in a spherical way that you do not hold your breath. Breathing in a full body has been practiced for millennia to enhance the capacity to relax and release energy blocks within the body/mind which improves happiness and saintly awareness.

Inhalation from Health Qigong, despite its appearance is comprised of four actions:

* Breathe deeply in

* Breathe deeply out

* Holding your breath (When you breathe in or hold the air that you breathe for a short amount of period of time is known as breath holding)

A breath gap (when you breath out and stop your breathing for a short time is known as breathing break during the process)

The entire process is what creates breath. The breath should be taken in one exhalation and then one blowout However, not every breath should include breath holding or breath gap. Breath gap and breath holding must be performed with a soft touch in accordance with the requirements of body movements, like when you stretch your limbs, if you are nervous about them, move your body or lift it or when you want to take an interruption or relax your mind.

Before you begin

Make sure you are in an area of calm where you are able to be unabated and free of distraction. Put your eyes shut for a couple of minutes in total surrender to your breath and no other beliefs.

How Do I Begin?

If you can, sit up straight If you can, sit in an upright-backed chair. You can feel the gentle shift of your tongue towards the gum line right at the rear of your front or top teeth.Let your shoulders ease and away from the neckline and allow your torso muscles relax down to the level of to your lower rib cage.

How to breathe in

As you breathe in, imagine breathing into your upper pelvis. Of obviously, your lungs will not necessarily go that far however, thinking about breathing into your higher pelvis will cause the lower lungs to fill first.And then , your upper body will surely expand too.

How to exhale

C.

When you exhale again, allowing your shoulders to sink and then relax towards your neckline. The air will be drained out of your upper part first.

D.

And then , you'll empty from your lower lungs while allowing your abdominal wall to gently move into the inside.

In a short time and when you're prepared slowly, and slowly, open your eyes. As you exhale to your mind, imagine the brain and let go of the thoughts fixed it's stuck on. It's as if your mind were a force that you've effortlessly. The mind is squeezed with no reason or reason at all, in the moment, you feel the airy fibres of your mind beginning to loosen, to expand out, and then to loosen to let this expanding lightness flow as you breathe in. If you allow your breath to take a deep breath from your peaceful body, it's like your brain is able to breathe and let go.

How do you finish

As soon as you awake, you can give yourself a couple of moments to lay around and soak in the deep-sea of happiness and joy that you've transformed into. Let yourself be lifted, bleached and open. Relax in this place of total security and total acceptance. Nothing to worry about and nothing to add into, you are eternally suspended in this place of elegance, revered and cherished because of who you are.

Caution

If your first experience with this Qigong breathing exercise didn't inspire your mind and alleviate your stress, then you should try it again, and not do it this time. The problems we encounter when using these methods aren't due to the fact that we weren't trying hard enough or weren't properly sufficiently trained, but usually because we try too much.

Inhaling too much and exhaling with a breath gaps could cause damage to your health. In the end the breath in and exhale should flow smoothly and slowly and without straining your body by inhaling at the top of your lungs and exhaling the entire amount you can. Breath-holding and breathing, pauses should be done in a relaxed manner. When you are doing this too often or using too much energy isn't good for your physical health.

Chapter 7: Qigong Simple Exercises For

Beginner

Qigong Exercise to help maintain a healthy body position and improve blood circulation

It is one of the most simple Qigong exercises, but it is possible to go as deep as you like. The basic idea is that we stir the body upwards and downwards by inhaling. We can use this Lao Gong point to center your brain, or move the brain to the entire length of the body, starting from the foot. In the second case approach, we're moving downwards through the foot and relaxing the body, through the breath, before dissolving, softening and calming the body by the exhalation.

The location of Lao Gong Point

In the middle of your palm in between the 3rd and 2nd metacarpal bones but close to the third, and in the area that moves the point of the middle of the finger, when a fist formed.

Benefits

The focus of the exercise is upon your Lao Gong point in the Centre of the palm. If you carry this practice across your entire body, you is energized, the blood circulation will be stronger and the flow is good for your heart, poor flow, arthritis. Additionally, it helps you to develop better physical health.

Standing positions

Relax and position yourself naturally by keeping your feet or shoulders wide between your shoulders.

* Allow your arms to rise above your body until they reach shoulder-height (breathing into).

Begin to lower your arms slowly till your hands the same height as your waist.

A bit of winding can help soften the knees (breathing out).

Exercise Tips

Do your best to avoid bending your knees backwards, and let your breathing determine your posture (rather than allowing your movement to direct your breathing). Move at a pace that is suitable for you.

Rainbow Dance

This is where we shift the weight and link the practice of plummeting and exhilarating along with exhalation. The palms form parallels to your eyes as well as the Bai Hui tip of the crown of the head. Also, we must keep the body in a single position, and to avoid distortion of the knees. Allow the underfoot to effectively "receive" the load.

Bai Hui Point is located. Bai Hui Point

The most important point is located near the apex of the head. It is located on the edge of the row that connects the apexes of both ears.

Steps

Stand calmly and logically with your feet a little wider than shoulder width away. Relax your right leg by putting all your weight on it.

* While you raise your left hand up to shoulder height, look at your open palm. Bring your right hand up, and hold it over the your head. Do this with your left hand. The Lao Gong point in front of your head, and that of the Bai Hui point.

Begin slowly shifting your weight from one (left) leg while you move your arms around in a typical circle over your head.

* Move to the right and then bend to the right and bend your left leg. Take your right hand to shoulder height , then look at it. Your left hand should be carried over your head and up to your head. Lao Gung point facing above your head. Then, look to you will be looking at the Bai Hui point.

Continue to blink between your right and left sides, while remaining regular and relaxed. (You may notice that your breathing becomes an elongated pattern as you ascend and out, or on the way down, based on the speed of your activity).

Note

There may be some numbness or pain in the arms and shoulders especially if you perform this exercise for only a brief duration. Try relaxing and softening any tension in order to assist in the release of any blockage of Qi.

Once you've figured out the motion, you can follow the gentle dance of this exercise while you shift your body weight from side to side. While focusing on the upper body, make sure to maintain a relationship with the earth through both of your feet . Also, avoid any incline or collapsing in your knees.

The Love and Healing Heart Energy

Draw your palms toward your centre Keep your right hand high , while your palm is facing the Earth and your left hand in the ground, facing the air, making the power ball.

Step 1 Step 1: Push to the left

* Twist your right palm facing ahead

* Exhale

* Turn your left hand left at 45 degrees and up to chest-high

Step 2 . Return to the Centre

* Revolve your right palm

• Twist the body from waist to your Centre

* As you inhale, the smoke, you should twitch your palms

* Bring your right hand towards the waist

* Right hand just in front of the space

* Left palm facing in the direction of Earth

Step 3 Move to the right

* Turn your left hand to the opposite side and then inwards

* Exhale

* Turn your left hand left at 45 degrees, and then up to the chest level.

4. Return back to the Centre

* Rotate your left palm

Then, twist your body around your waist towards the Centre

* When you inhale, twist your palms

* Bring your left hand towards your waist

* Left hand in between the spaces

Right hand facing the Earth

Note: Must repeat 6 times

Chapter 8: Enhance Your Focus By Using Horse

Posture Technique

Steps

Then, slow down your body and mind. If you're performing this exercise for the first time, create (or create) an energizing and peaceful setting.

Horse Stance

Let's look at the horse's posture

A horse-like posture for martial arts. Any posture can be used. Maintain the position for around one or more minutes and this could increase the effects of the subsequent steps. If you're extremely weak, then you could skip this step.

Get out of the horse standing stance and get up immediately. Reset your body and your mind. Your academic, physical or emotional stress will sour your compassion and affect your performance in the following step. Massage your hands together for a couple of minutes. Keep your eyes closed.

Then move your palms toward the opposite direction like you are pressing the surface of a small beach ball. Imagine the chi connecting in your palms. Moving your hands at a rate of 1-3 squeezes per second, over the range of 6 to 24 inches. Keep this up for 2-4 minutes, or as long as necessary, until you notice the sensation of your hands. There may be the sensation of heat, itching, vibrating or a strong, compelling attraction. A lot of people experience these sensations on their first training session; some will need repeating training every day until they achieve a desired result.

Return to the Centre

Step forward with the right foot. for balance

Scoop of water from the ocean

Go to the right

* Shift mass until you have a precise foot

* Turn around at the waist and draw both arms downwards , and then towards the right knee.

* Cross your hands across the right-hand lap

* Palms visage upwards

* Top of skull is aligned with the right foot.

Clean up

* Transfer the weight to the left leg.

* Slowly straighten your body straight

* Inhale slowly

* Keep your hands crossed over your head.

Separate hands:

* Arms can be split and expanded up and out

* Palms are viewed from the ground.

* Exhale

You must repeat the process 6 times.

Chapter 9: Three Treasures: The Essential To

Health And Well-Being

In Traditional Chinese Medicine, and particularly in the field of Qigong, there's an important concept that can be understood to comprehend our health, which in turn affects our overall well-being and the our quality of life.

We discuss "The three treasures of health".

In conventional theories, they can be described in a poetic and metaphorical manner.

It is important to realize the fact that these theories were created over time in a historical and social setting that is quite different from our present.

So, how they share their knowledge could at times be quite unexpected.

The three treasures have been extensively researched and utilized in Chinese medicine , and we are able to discover a myriad of writings which go into greater detail about the meaning behind them.

Yet at the same we're discussing an idea that on an elementary level is simple and easy to grasp and can be used as an initial basis for creating regimens for taking medical treatment of our bodies.

According to traditional Chinese medicine , the human body is composed of three components: the physical body, energy, and the mind.

In other words, we can categorize the composition of the human being into three categories: mental, energetic, and physical and each of them will correspond to the various precious stones (jing Jing , qi Qi Shen Shen).

1. The physical body is all that we can view and touch.It encompasses the whole body, from the skin to internal organs, traversing through bones, muscles tendons...

This portion is related to the JING (Jing) that is commonly described as the essence, that is the primary substance of our body, being the base material of all of its tissues. It is a result of its manifestation in the physical body.

The strength of our constitution is dependent on the jing we have; the strength of jing can be seen as a healthy and strong body. Contrarily weak jings will result in problems with physical weakness, growth and so on.

2. The energetic part of us; it's something that we can't perceive, or even touch but that we do sense: in a way it gives us life as well as allows the physical parts to perform. It's what Chinese refer to as QI (pronounced Chi) (Qi) (generally translated as "energy").

The qi moves through a number of channels, known as JIN-LOU which allows it to flow to every body part. In Chinese medical treatment, there are various kinds of qi, based on their source, function, or place of origin. Different functions are associated with it, like heating, propulsion, defense and so on.

3. The mind is the one that controls the Qi (energy) to ensure that the Jing (body) can perform its function.

This means that it is our mind's action that controls the bodily functions by directing energy, whether consciously or in a state of unconscious. It's what the Chinese refer to as"SHEN (Shen) (often described to mean "spirit", "mind" or "consciousness").
Shen is a broad and broad word that is not limited to our mental activities, but also to the various physical manifestations of our vitality like expression, gaze, or any other general aspect.

We comprise mind, body, and energy. It is clear that all three aspects can be subdivided into numerous segments; the body is divided into different systems and there are various types of energy, and the mental part can be split into unconscious, conscious and so on.

The basic concept is that anything we're made of is possible to be part of any of these three areas.

A case study will allow us comprehend the meaning of the concepts.

Let's concentrate upon one part of the arm. It is the physical part. It is visible and felt.

Let's move it. To do this, we require something we can't see or feel, but we can feel. This is the energy or qi.

Also, we need something to give us the authority to carry out the action that is our brain or shen.

Thus, we already observe in this case that the three components will always be connected My mind (shen) transmits the energy (qi) towards the arm (jing) in order to allow it to move.

In reality, jing, Qi and shen are all terms can be analyzed and explained in a more comprehensive and complete manner. But the most important thing is to comprehend that in a an extremely general and fundamental way the human body is composed of these three elements.

If we are able to focus and improve each of them the health of our body and life , will be more enjoyable.

It is crucial to realize how the treasures cannot work in isolation.

Our entire body is an entire unit, and we can't separate the functions of one component without impacting the rest of the body.

The practice of each one will affect the others and, as a the principle of most Qigong systems, all three treasures have to be coordinated for our practice to produce the desired outcomes.

We know today all that exists in the Universe is energy and nothingness. This means that we live in a vibratory world in which everything originates from the same source. It manifests in various ways based on the nature or frequency.

This is in line with the old Chinese concept of qi which suggests that this qi energy runs through all that is within the universe.

Condensing it, it transforms into matter, and once it has been clear, it transforms into spirit. Everything vibrates and lives thanks to the qi which flows through it.

From this perspective The three treasures, or three dimensions that we separate the human being are in fact three different manifestations of the identical "life power" and whatever else we choose to define it. It is for this reason that they must always be in harmony and a lot of our wellbeing will depend on the health of our body, mind and minds moving in the same direction.

Let's see what strategies we can use to accomplish this.

Chapter 10: Getting Started With Qigong

The benefits of qigong will make you want to learn it. You'll be pleased to know that practicing qigong can be simple. You don't need any expensive equipment. Before you can practice qigong, you should master three mindful alignments. First, the alignment that you learn is designed for the body, while the second alignment is for breathing and the third one is for the mind.

Although qigong is regarded as an exercise, it's more of a meditative experience. The emphasis is not on repetition. It is more the deliberate application of three deliberate adjustments: to increase the depth of the breath, stretch your spine and then to visualize healing or to clear the mind.

First Alignment: Control and adjust your movement or the Posture of Your Body

You can stand or sit up straight or spread your arms out. Imagine a connection that lifts your head towards the sky. Next, visualize a connection that connects your sacrum towards the earth's central. The upward and downward pull open the body's central point and fills it up with life-force energy.

The alignment of the spine creates spaces between vertebrae. This assists in releasing nerve compression , which can cause pain or discomfort. Posture adjustments allow organs to have the space they require to perform their functions optimally. The alignment is also beneficial to the circulation of blood and lymphatic fluids.

Second Mindful Alignment Relax and Refine Your Breath

Breath is the most essential instrument to activate the body's healing and revitalizing resources and to draw life force energy. Breathing is also the most simple to master. Inhale slowly with your nostrils. Breathe for the duration of one 1,000; two one thousand; three one thousand. Breaths should be slow, relaxed and slow, but not too fast. Relax even more when you exhale.

Third Mindful Alignment Awaken Your Mind

An old saying states that energy disperses when you are distracted by your thoughts. For the duration you want or for a short period, concentrate your mind on things that are simple like a flowing river of water and the sky with gentle floating clouds, or waves crashing upon the shore. Take a break and don't focus on the past or the future. Be present or aware by observing what you are doing, what you're feeling and where you are.

After you've completed the three conscious alignments, you can smile at yourself. The smile stimulates the limbic regions of the brain that - along alongside the brain's neural structure are linked to emotional behaviour. This helps to stimulate the chemistry in the brain to create feelings of wellbeing.

A right Kind of Qigong

Dong Qigong is among the methods to strengthen your overall health and to invest in your future wellbeing, health and overall health. But, it is important to understand that it is an 'period of exploration and discovery. The practitioner must be exposed to various styles and teachers before they is able to find the best one to suit their specific requirements. Furthermore, you need to know precisely what your purpose is while practicing Qigong.

Find a style or practice that will help you reach your goals. Different results are a result of different methods. Be sure to choose an qigong technique that can assist you in reaching the desired outcome. Certain forms of qigong include, for instance, the unique ability of developing sensory capabilities such as visual or olfactory.

Some qigong styles are focused on alleviate anxiety and soothe your nervous system. Certain forms of qigong will increase your mental clarity or endurance, while some support digestive function or immunity.

Learn, play and try out different styles of qigong as you improve and develop your own qigong style. Then, you will know that the qigong practice you'll be practicing is the best one for you. You can create your own collection of Qigong forms, and then introduce new movements and forms when you continue to practice.

Best Time to Qigong

Qigong is a practice that's typically done during the morning hours as it is the ideal timing since qi is the 'best and air pollution is typically minimal, and routines haven't begun to take over. Based on your personal preferences and your experiences, you may take a few minutes or 10 minutes, 30 minutes, or an hour. But, you should only practice qigong at the time that feels appropriate for you.

The question of when is the best time to practice Qigong is subjective and unclear. It's completely dependent on the practitioner, and some times might be more appropriate than others. There are guidelines based on the qigong style you're practicing However, it is best to incorporate qigong in your routine and practice regularly.

Qigong isn't something you can do at the beginning of the day and be stressed at work. All you need to do is to stop breathing, take a deep breath, and let your mind go. Do not practice qigong because you believe you need to do it, as it might simply be something you must do - as exercise. To ensure your safety and facilitate it to practice it in the early morning. Be mindful throughout the day, and you'll be in good shape.

Qigong and the Side Effects

You might be wondering if the Qigong practice causes adverse negative effects. There is no evidence to suggest that it causes side effects. In the case of a small number of people, adverse effects could be considered to be an exception. There are however, certain people who believe that the practice of energy medicine like qigong could cause adverse effects.

The Oriental Medical Doctor (OMD) might suggest that the only people that experience these effects could have mental issues prior to when they started practicing Qigong. The possibility of suffering negative effects of qigong might be very low in these individuals. There are others who claim that some advanced practices of qigong could cause issues such as obscure male sexual abstinence methods. But, these claims aren't proven.

Qigong is generally secure and there are no adverse effects as a result of it. Talk to an authorised qigong expert and learn more about the subject before you embark on your new journey.

Qigong Exercises

The practice of qigong will help you move, work and feel more energetic in your body. Qigong, though it appears unassuming, is an effective way to be more aware and alive. Qigong is only starting to gain traction in the West and there are many instructors and styles including definitions and definitions of the practice. The exercises are far too numerous to cover.

If you are just beginning qigong, it is important to build a strong base. Sets of qigong such as dragons, tigers and gates of energy, heaven and earth were developed by establishing a solid foundation in the mind. Each set of qigong focuses on specific internal elements such as body alignments breathing in and out, closing and opening fluids movement, moving stagnant energy.

Certain qigong systems make people more aware through improving your inner awareness and activating the meridians for acupuncture and moving Qi. Five sets of qigong relate to five different elements of water, fire, metal earth, wood and fire. The qigong exercises, that can be self-healing, help you to:

Rejuvenate and strengthen the brain's nervous system.

Feel and increase your Qi for health and fitness.

* Develop the sensitivity and depth to become a Qigong energy healer , or a qigong teacher.

Water Element (Energy Gates)

The 3,000-year-old self-healing qigong practice is designed intended for people who want to know more about different types of energy work like qigong or Tai Chi. It will teach you the fundamentals of the techniques to activate and harness qi to boost your health, counteract aging's effects, and decrease stress. Energy Gates qigong will aid in integrating and practicing internal power elements (neigong) such as breathing, dissolving spinal activation, aligning and shifting weight.

Energy Gates consists of six sequenced actions:

* Standing in three sections scan, dissolve, and sinking your Qi.

* Cloud Hands

*The First Swing

* Second Swing

* Third Swing

*The Taoist Spine Stretch

Energy Gates teaches you to maintain your body's alignment to effortlessly shift weight as you move your body and to breathe for longevity. These are all essential to achieve a healthy, energetic lifestyle that is more crucial than keeping your appearance good and healthy.

Energy Gates' core element is standing up for at least 15 minutes each day. The neigong method helps to build Qi in your body, improves consciousness within you, and allows you know where qi is blocked. As you begin, you will be able to imagine your body with your mind. Begin with high up in your head and move towards your feet. This will help you be aware of your body and to ease into your body.

As you practice and progress you will be able to utilize your mind's intent to release the blockage of qi and unlock the major energy gates of your body. When the flow of qi begins flowing freely through your body, you'll feel more energized. Energy Gates is among the most effective Qigong set for internal use to increase energy levels and relieving your nerves.

Wood Element (Heaven and Earth)

Heaven as well as Earth is an exercise that is simple and repetitive to increase the flow of your qi. It can help treat back and spine injuries. It is also effective especially in reducing the effects of carpal tunnel syndrome as well as RSI (repetitive injuries to the body).

Heaven as well as Earth is an evocative of Taoist Qi Arts, but it's not enough to take over your life. It is a perfect example of how qigong works:

* Protest you internal.

• Open your mind for new ideas.

You will not be bored while you practice.

Heaven and Earth's fundamental motion is Circling Hands that can be seamlessly integrated into tai-chi's basic movements, particularly when it is done by using changes in weight, waist turns and three basic circles. This allows beginners to comprehend tai-chi a little however in a digestible and concise method.

Heaven and Earth's basic actions are receptacles to internal qi energy work. Learn how you can open or close joint (pulsing) without using muscle tension. Closing and releasing is an essential energetic process that connects Heaven as well as Earth. It allows you to move Qi through the acupuncture meridian lines, fascia and joints in the body as well as manage the ascending and descended Qi flow. The body's ability of spring and be able to pulse with an elastic quality is an essential element of neigong's energetic practice.

Heaven and Earth's more advanced levels will help you energetically open and close the soft and hard tissues of the body and cavities and move on to closing and opening the areas of your subtle anatomy (aura points, points as well as channels). Internal components can be integrated into other practices of energy and are essential for Taoist practices which are more advanced.

Metal Element (Bend the Bow)

As a sophisticated qigong system, Bend the Bow focuses on strengthening and regenerating the spine. The set of qigong integrates components of neigong to manage the spine's energy. The Qigong set teaches the user in advanced neigong components that aid in strengthening the spine, replenish and manage the spine's qi energy and treat back issues that are severe, such as the scoliosis.

Bend and Bow enables you to regulate the vertebrae's individual movements that aren't considered as possible within Western medicine.

1. The initial phase loosens and warms the spine and helps relax your nervous system.

2. In the second stage you will learn the basic reverse breathing techniques as well as physical movements will allow you to control your spine energy.

3. The third phase lets you to:

You can simultaneously open and close all of your spinal vertebrae to form an integral unit.

Together, the internal organs' energy and physical movements to joints and spine.

* The space between each spinal vertebra.

* Manage the flow of fluids around the spinal cord and your brain.

* Move each vertebra independently at any time in any direction, without physical motion.

• Be mindful of correcting right and left imbalances in your body as well as in your spinal vertebrae.

Fire Element (Spiraling Energy Body)

Spiraling Energy Body lets you increase your energy levels . You are also able to master the flow of qi through circles and spirals throughout your body. Spiraling Energy Body helps you improve the speed at that qi moves through the body. It can be beneficial for meditation and can be utilized to redirect a tense mind into paths that are steady.

Spiraling Energy Body is energetically and emotionally demanding and should be taught after having gained a solid understanding of the physical and energetic aspects that open your Body's Energy Gates. You should only test Spiraling Energy Body after getting an understanding of the dissolving and standing techniques.

Then you will receive the custom-designed standing posture according to your body's particular energetics at your manifested Qi development level. The customized posture could assist you in addressing an illness you might or might have or to enhance your hidden abilities or energy potential in your own life.

The neighing aspects of the Spiraling Energy Body permit you to:

* Project qi along your spiraling pathways.

* Direct upward flow of energy.

* Send or release energy at will from to any body part.

* neutralizing and changing negative energy.

* Enable your central, right, and left channels. Then, activate the microcosmic orbit.

Earth Element (Gods Playing in the Clouds)

Gods In the Clouds includes the most potent and earliest Taoist rejuvenation methods. It is the only Qigong Liu Hung Chieh (Taoist Lineage Master) used to increase longevity past the age of 50. It enhances the energetic, breathing and physical elements of early qigong practices.

Engaging in Gods' Play in the cloud can rid the body of negative energy. It can strengthen your bones as well as stabilize and open up your central energy channel and the heart center to energize your brain and remove spiritual blockages. It also enhances the breathing, energy and physical aspects of the primary qigong programmes. It is also the final step in integrating the neigong's elements and is the final phase of learning how to improve and balance the energy of the back, spine and the three tantiens.

Gods playing in the clouds could be a spiritual connection with Taoist meditation.

Qigong Tui Na Energy Healing

Qigong Energy Healing (qigong Tui Na) is an Chinese medicine branch designed to release, balance, and open up qi within other people. It is possible to release energy through your eyes, your voice, and hands to aid in healing. In order to be able to heal others, you need to first be able to liberate and open your own qi. You must be aware of the pathways that your qi moves.

Understanding Qigong Energy Healing is a matter of when you build a solid foundation in qigong to gain the ability to sense an awareness of your own qi prior to manipulating other people's qi. The most important aspect of training in Qigong Energy Therapy involves knowing the regenerative Qi methods that help you avoid being spiritually, emotionally, and physically exhausted while treating other people's Qi.

The principle of Qigong is, if you have to spend an amount of time with patients you must spend a quarter of the time practicing techniques to regenerate to avoid burning out.

Qigong and Nutrition

The qigong exercise you do with the intention of balancing your body's internal balance could be counterproductive if you additionally counter the practice by eating foods that are not 'credible' in nutritional value. The food you consume is an essential factor in your mood. The feeling of wellbeing and health is based on the food choices you consume. About 70% of your immunity comes from food. Therefore, if you're sick, take note of the food you are eating and decide what should be altered.

Food can be a bridge to the cells in your body and can let you know how important it is to you. Food is also the first chance to fight off illness and is also the first step to help heal your body. Foods that are unhealthy can cause you to be tired, slow and even cause illness. The importance of nutrition, besides being about feeling good, it is also the foundation and the basis from which all other aspects of your life are derived from.

Qigong and healthy nutrition go hand-in-hand. There are many ways to do qigong, there are many different ways to make sure you are balancing your nutritional needs and Qigong. Here are some suggestions and guidelines in balancing nutrition and qigong.

Salads are Good

The Western diet's main ingredient is salad. When compared to traditional Chinese stir-fry method for preparing vegetable, fresh, healthy salad is an enjoyable and healthier option. But, if you suffer from an 'emaciated stomach' it is not recommended to take a salad.

Iced drinks accumulate Damp Qi

It's a bad habit to regularly drink iced drinks such as iced tea, iced tea, Iced juice and coke with ice. Ice is known to drain the stomach's energy and could result in damp qi, or cold qi to remain inside the body. This could lead to obesity.

Too Much dessert and cheese Could make Qi sticky.

One of the weaknesses that is a part of Western food system is over consumption of cheese and desserts and other dairy products, which make the body's Qi unclear and sticky. Consequently, it slows the flow of qi. Smoking can also make a person's Qi filthy.

As Taoist classics say, "Five colors make the eyes blind, five tastes render the tongue dumb and five sounds leave people blind." Five is a sign of imbalance or excessive. In qigong it is best to consume light meals rather than eating a lot of delicious and heavy meals.

toasted food and Barbecue Cause 'Too Much Smoke'

Many Westerners are fond of eating toasty and oven-baked food as well as barbecue. These meals, unfortunately, are brimming with "fire" or yin. To balance it take care to eat these foods in moderation.

Spiritualists Should also eat clean food

Dietary requirements for people who are normal and spiritual practitioner differ. Tai chi is a spiritual practice or yoga can connect the practitioner with spiritual energy. The common feature of spiritual energies is that spiritualists favor healthy and vegetarian food.

If you are a qigong practitioner for every day for an hour it is not advised with your Qigong practices. It can reduce the power of your practice, and can cause serious health problems. Another example is onion that is beneficial to people who are not ill. But a practitioner of qigong might find that onion is too stimulating for their Qi. Onion can affect the harmony and smoothness of the Qi.

Cleaning is a great way to Enhance the taste of your food

Many people are aware that certain foods are which are unhealthy However, they lack the motivation to control their appetites. Certain people are also conscious of their food choices to the point of obsessing. It is beneficial that when Qigong sessions they experience a change in their taste and their bodies are more clean. The bodies of those who practice qigong generally choose clean and vegetarian food. Therefore, cleansing is an excellent way to gain an excellent flavor.

The Taoist "No Food Wisdom: Bigu

After years of practice qigong the practitioner can attain the 'too qi-filled for eating the food. This is known as bigu, that literally means "avoid grains. Bigu is a specialized practice of qigong for cleansing basics. Also known as energized fasting and energized fasting, the bigu method - which is built on the universal energy precondition - differs from the 'food-forbidden therapy.'

Practitioners of Bigu may not feel hungry or might feel a slight sense of hunger. The effects of Bigu's detoxification are amazing and can lead to the process of rejuvenation. To reach the bigu state however, that you must engage in many years of Qigong practices.

Acid-Alkaline vs. Yin-Yang

Western nutritionists are aware of the alkaline and acid characteristics of fooditems, however many people aren't aware of the significance of Yin-Yang characteristics in foods. There are many people who have various levels of imbalance in Yin Yang that can cause various ailments. For instance, some people are prone to heat, and others can easily become cold. Food choices can help ease the discomfort or worsen it.

Ginseng is an example. It is widely believed to be an effective nutritional supplement. However, certain types of ginseng are Yin and others are Yang depending on the location the Ginseng is produced. In the end, a healthy diet needs to be developed specifically for a person's Yin-Yang balance.

There is no Aura In Fast Food

Fast food restaurants are commonplace throughout many Western countries. Fast food chains are increasing in other parts around the globe, and even in China. The issue is whether fast food really is rubbish. Many people believe that refrigeration helps keep food bacteria at bay Therefore fast food is an odious and efficient method to make food in large quantities.

Quigong instructors and practitioners who are experienced However, they have the capacity to recognize that meat patties don't have any aura', which means they lack essential clean energy. It doesn't matter whether you consume fast food in moderation however, if you eat lots of it, then toxins could be accumulating slowly inside your body and illness can sneak in.

In qigong, as well as eating it is important to maintain balance. If you're not a serious practitioner , and If you're practicing Qigong for the sake of staying well-balanced and healthy it's not doing any harm to consume Western foods , but in moderate amounts. It is possible to eat fast food or junk food, but only sparingly. It's okay to have a cold beverage every at least once in a while. It is also essential to incorporate healthy salads into your diet. In the end, you'll achieve the perfect balance between doing qigong and eating healthy. This balance will allow you to get a healthier body and spiritual awareness.

Chapter 11: Health Benefits From Qigong

In the last couple of years, more experts have begun to advocate Qigong as a treatment for a variety of medical ailments. The increasing popularity is growing. Qigong has spread across the boundaries of China as more and more practitioners from all over the Western world have begun to recommend it to treat high blood pressure and atherosclerosis, as well as digestive disorders including the ulcers of the peptic. Studies have proven that those suffering from chronic liver disease and obesity, diabetes or both are able to benefit from regular exercise of Qigong. Studies have also proved its efficacy for women who are entering menopausal and those who suffer from insomnia or burnout, or have abnormal sleeping routines (insomnia). Qigong may have an anti-cancer effect , and can be a great help for other chronic illnesses like the fibromyalgia or cervical spondylosis. It aids in reducing different kinds of pain, including lower back pain and leg pain. It's effective for patients suffering from issues with the eyes (for instance myopia, for example).).

The most significant benefit that Qigong can provide is the fact that it promotes peace to the body and mind. It can have a positive effect on circulation, enhancing the flow of blood in tiny blood vessels, and protecting them with no excessive contractions. The benefits of Qigong on circulation have resulted in doctors recommending Qigong for ailments like chest angina as well as for migraines that are chronic. If you have a patient with circulatory issues like Raynaud's Syndrome the routine practice of Qigong can provide a substantial improvement in symptoms. Qigong assists in restoring health, assisting the patient to get rid of tension or discomfort. One of the most significant advantages is that it keeps blood pressure in check. In addition studies have shown that it may lower blood pressure in people who suffer from hypertension.

Whatever their age people who are able to practice Qigong consistently claim to are more energetic. This may be due with the reality that Qigong is recognized as an effective booster of the immune system. It appears that Qigong can protect your body from diverse types of illnesses by targeting the antigens in an effective manner. Through boosting immunity, Qigong is also a shield against various types of cancer. In essence, Qigong works by improving the function of various system of the body - particularly the cardiovascular, neurological and circulatory systems, as well as respiratory digestion, and lymphatic ones.

Qigong is recommended for those who suffer from chronic illnesses like it was previously mentioned. As an example, Qigong has been shown to be extremely effective for those diagnosed with fibromyalgia. It helps in alleviating symptoms and enhancing the overall level of functioning. In terms of cardiovascular health, Qigong has been found to lower your resting heart rate, and also the amount in bad cholesterol (thus protecting from atherosclerosis). Regarding breathing, Qigong has many benefits, because it reduces the rate of respiration and enhances the exchange of gasses in the lungs. It's also been found to be extremely beneficial in managing symptoms of patients identified with asthma, or irritation of the bronchi (bronchitis).

The continuous practice of Qigong can have a positive physical impact on the brain, increasing blood flow to the cortex , and decreasing the chance of having strokes. Studies conducted with epilepsy patients have shown that Qigong is a viable option to decrease the frequency and intensity of epileptic seizures. This has enabled medical doctors and other experts to utilize Qigong for other neurological disorders that are characterised, along with other signs by seizures. In relaxing the brain's structures, Qigong has also helped sufferers with abnormal sleep routines or insomnia. It is believed that by assisting the brain to get into a state deep sleep, insomnia sufferers are able to attain the peace of mind required for rest.

While Qigong isn't only a form of exercise for the body It is worth noting that it has an impact on the muscles and skeletal system. In addition to improving posture and body balance it also helps to strengthen muscles and improve the flexibility of joints. For those who have sustained various injuries or went through a surgical procedure, Qigong is the best way to manage the pain and restore normal function. Qigong is a method of exercise that Qigong can also help those suffering from chronic or acute inflammation in joints, enhancing the function and decreasing the discomfort caused by the inflammation.

Concerning mental well-being, Qigong has been shown to decrease the stress that is associated with burnout. Furthermore, Qigong can improve the symptoms of those suffering from anxiety or other obsessive-compulsive disorders. Continuous practice of Qigong can have a positive impact on the mood of a person and reduces the symptoms that are associated with depression, and creating an atmosphere where there is a feeling of joy (balances emotional states). In addition it is believed that Qigong will improve memory, as well as other similar cognitive functions.

The anti-cancer effects of Qigong is backed through the elimination of free radicals that are play a major role in the degradation of the various tissues. Qigong is being more frequently used to speed up healing process for a broad range of medical issues which include injuries resulting from various accidents, or as a post-operative treatments. It is also suggested to those working in a sedentary position because it improves their posture and builds up the muscles.

The positive impact of Qigong on the health of bones has been demonstrated in numerous research studies. When women are entering menopausal, Qigong reduces the bone loss and increases the risk of fractures. In addition it helps improve bone health by improving the overall bone mineral density. Due to its association with physical exercise, Qigong is also recommended for those who have BMIs above 30, as an effective way to fight overweight.

The list of health-enhancing effects that Qigong can bring to the body is long. As you can see it is able to lower blood pressure as well as improve the efficiency that the respiratory organs perform. Research has proven that it regulates hormone levels, which improves the function of kidneys and the sexual libido (patients say they have greater sexual vitality or energy). It also has an impact on mental health and can improve the sight and hearing, and it helps keep the skin healthy and elastic (helps by removing the toxins and improves your appearance). Overall, Qigong guarantees an improved quality of life . It's interesting enough for those who are healthy, but as well in those suffering from chronic diseases.

Chapter 12: Qigong Practice

Qigong can be practiced in a variety of method, but all methods have the same goal and it is to bring the body into alignment with breath and the mind. Modern Qigong practices incorporate meditation in two forms - still and moving still - as well as massage and physical manipulation as well as chanting and meditation using the use of sound, as well as non-contact treatments and various external agents. They also require people to adopt various poses, and work their magic in cultivating and balancing the Qi or vital energy.

In accordance with the level of intensity in the practice, Qigong is classified into two broad types. On the one hand, you can find the energetic or active Qigong practiced on slow movements that appear to flow (this is often referred to by the name dong gong). In contrast, you can find the meditative, passive form of Qigong that is built around a posture still and focusing on breathing as well as its inner movement (more generally referred to as jing Gong). Based on the external intervention Qigong is a practice that Qigong is classified as internal and external. In the first instance the treatment is provided by the Qigong practitioner, the person trying to direct the flow of Qi to the person receiving the treatment. Within the inner Qigong the individual practices self-healing and balances the qi by himself.

The practice of meditation that is based on movement is frequently chosen by people who are fascinated by Qigong as it is an underlying principle of the slow , flowing movements described earlier and also on breath (the breathing is rhythmic, deep , and typically diaphragmatic rather than abdominal). Moving meditation helps practitioners of Qigong practitioner to find the peace of mind, and to imagine how Qi, or life energy, is directed throughout the body.

Moving meditation is a part of the lively exercise in Qigong The movements that are part of the practice are usually performed with the highest level of focus. This is due to the fact that all Qigong exercises must be controlled by the breath and the mind and help the person performing them become more conscious on both a physical as well as a mental level. In certain regions of China It is normal to perform these slow movements in order to mimic the movements of animals.

Physically it is a dynamic exercise. Qigong is an exercise that is beneficial for the body. As these slow motions are practiced frequently it strengthens the muscles and joints get strengthened and the individual is no longer stiff or rigid. The practice helps get various bodily fluids flowing, whether talking about lymph, blood as well as the synovial liquid inside joints. The people who have tried the dong gong claim the improvement in their posture and also their proprioception which was evident within a short time as they became more aware of the space their bodies are in and how their body moves in the space.

There are plenty of people who favor an approach that is static like Qigong by embracing a broad variety of still postures for a certain amount of time, and focusing on the breathing. In many ways it is similar to the practice that's static. Qigong is comparable to yoga, because both require the use of various poses, along with a attention to breathing.

The balance and development of the qi is believed to be among the greatest advantages of the meditation practice Qigong. This intricate practice requires intense concentration on breathing and at the same time by focusing on the qi in the whole body. Other components that are essential to the practice are the mantras, shifting and the focus on the sound. They all work together to bring the focus of meditation to a point at which one is focusing solely on the flow of Qi.

Qigong is founded on a number of general principles, which end up are useful for guiding the actual practice. One of the main concepts is motion. As already stated, Qigong is based on moves that are executed in a controlled and slow method. The choreography of these moves frequently creates the impression of flowing. The breathing pattern is the second key principle of Qigong Practitioners are instructed to concentrate on deep and diaphragmatic breathing in accordance with a certain rhythm. This rhythm is vital in that it allows breathing to be in sync with the movement of various bodily fluids.

Awareness is another important principle of Qigong It is believed that by entering the state of meditation one can attain peace, as well as physical and mental awareness. In Qigong you'll see that these principles connect in the most fascinating manner. Meditation can lead not just to calmness and consciousness but also allows those who are a Qigong practitioner to pay attention to the flow of energy within the body. Chanting is among the main principles of Qigong practice because it gives one the opportunity to focus on the sound in the process of meditation.

When you practice Qigong There are many aspects that will allow you to reap the most benefits. For instance, if fix your eyes at a single spot and focus on it, you'll be able to attain an elongated mindset. If you keep your spine straight and your feet planted to the ground you'll be able to maintain the poses during stationary practice for longer durations of time. If you concentrate on your breathing, you'll notice that your muscles and joints are relaxed, allowing you to experience a new state of calm. If you are more calm and relaxed, feel more relaxed, the easier it is to direct the qi through the body. When you are relaxed, you will be able to rid your mind from unnecessary thoughts and experience an awareness state. When you have mastered the art of Qigong you'll have achieved the state of total stillness.

Chapter 13: Exercises In Qigong To Aid In Self-

Healing

There are many Qigong exercises which can be done to help you heal yourself aiding you in achieving an attitude of joy and success in every endeavor that you begin. Remember that these exercises can aid in balancing and developing your Qi.

Sitting Qigong

It is a sitting Qigong exercises are usually performed in the morning to provide the required relaxation needed for the remainder days. The benefit of these workouts is the fact that they are able to be performed by people suffering from various ailments who are bedridden or in a position that makes it difficult to stand for long durations of time.

One of the most simple exercises to perform while sitting Qigong exercises, which is recommended for those who are new to the practice, is closing your eyes while sitting. The best position that is recommended for the exercise involves to sit with the legs crossed and your attention solely upon your solar plexus. You must let your body relax completely to feel as if it were flowing. The hands are placed in the lap , and the spine is kept in a relaxed position. The breathing is steady and consistent, while your thoughts are cleared of all thoughts that are not necessary. When you've taken the position you want, you must to sit still and focus for at minimum five minutes. It is possible to increase the length of your practice on a regular basis.

Hands on the Head

A great exercise to practice self-healing is that where the hands are held over the head. The exercise can be divided into two sections - for the first one it is necessary to tap your teeth for about thirty-six times. The suggestion is to consume the saliva produced during the process. The tapping of your teeth is aimed at stimulating the qi gums' level. as a result it is not just that tooth decay prevented, but also the teeth's roots are strengthened. Additionally the tapping of teeth can affect the brain cavity, assisting you to get your mind clear.

The second portion of the exercise will require you placing your hands together, and putting them on the side to your skull. The next step is to push your body and head to the back using your hands to counteract (forward in the direction of forward). It is necessary to repeat this exercise 9 times, taking deep breaths while pulling, and exhaling in the relaxation phase. This exercise can have amazing effects on your health, and can help you straighten your spine, and to improve circulation of the Qi in the back region and, consequently, to reduce back discomfort. It can also be used to boost lung capacity because it requires coordination of breathing and the movements you are doing.

Clear you mind

If you're in search of an exercise that will help you get your mind off of things, the next exercise is ideal for you. The first step is to sit on your feet with the legs cross. You then covering your ears using your hands with your fingers spread wide apart. The placement of your fingers is crucial since you have to place your middle fingers just below the protuberance of the occipital. The next step in the exercise is to position your index fingers above the middle one, applying pressure on your head. The exercise should be repeated for 24 times which will result in the development of a sound that drums in the brain's cavity. You may not be aware of this, but the sound of drumming helps get your mind clear efficiently.

Standing Qigong

Standing exercises are fundamental to the Qigong practice and are suggested to people who are competent to stand in such postures (no prior conditions that would cause difficulty in standing). Beginners should begin with the Qigong practice by standing as long as they are able to, for at least 15 minutes each day. This will help to increase being aware of your own body, and aids in the flow of the qi within the body. It also helps the practitioner determine whether there is any blockage or not. For those who are new to the practice begin with your mind to look around your body. start from the top, and then perform slow scanning to your feet. In time, you'll be relaxed and more conscious of the events going on within your body.

Another excellent stand Qigong exercise is that of hands that are cloudy. It is possible to begin this exercise by taking the proper posture standing with your feet separated and your spine straight. put your chin into a position and then relax your entire body. Your knees should be bent slightly, making it easier to relax. Then, you can begin doing slow-motion moves in various directions and shift you body weight from one side to the next. The purpose of this workout is moving your arms in such a way that they are in sync with your entire body, thereby promoting the flow of qi.

Three Swings

The three swings exercise designed for people who wish to improve the flow of qi throughout the entire body and have a positive impact on internal organs. The name of the exercise reveals that you must take three different swings with your arms. Each one has distinct benefits for health. The first one is believed to stimulate the qi of the internal organs situated in lower abdominal. It has an effect that is beneficial to the urogenital region, but also on the stomach as well as the intestines. The second one will positively impact organs like the liver, spleen and the pancreas. It can also be practiced to heal the adrenal glands and ensuring their functioning. Third swings are designed to the lungs, the heart and the brain. It also can have a positive impact on the spine, ensuring the correct space between vertebrae, and also preventing degeneration of the discs of the vertebrae.

These are only a few Qigong exercises to be used to begin your Qigong practice. Once you become a regular participant of Qigong you will learn numerous other exercises that have benefits to your health.

Chapter 14: Important Things To Keep In Mind

About Qigong And The Practices Of Qigong

When you begin to become a regular practitioner of Qigong There are certain aspects you'll be required to consider. The most crucial aspects is these gates of energy, being the points that are where the balance of Qi actually occurs. The concept of balancing qi is a long-standing tradition that dates back to the beginning of China and is as relevant in the present as it was when it was. Regularly practicing Qigong can help you feel the energy channels throughout your body. As you clear your mind of all thoughts and enter into a state of relaxation, you'll discover how to feel these points and enhance the flow of Qi.

Through the entire human body there exist a variety of energy gates that you'll learn to recognize when you exercise Qigong. The most significant energies gates, or areas are the The crown of the head, the eyes and the ears (their central point) temples, as well as the jaw (four points within the jaw by itself). In the mouth is another energy gate that is located in the area where your tongue almost touches the palate. The skull's base and the spaces between the cervical vertebrae, and the shoulders are also considered energy gates. They continue to be present found in the wrists, elbows and hands. Soon you will realize most of them are in joints, like the sterno-costal joint , or the costal-vertebral joint. This listing of Qigong points is further enriched through the solar-plexus hip sockets, and belly. Lower abdomen those energy gateways are situated at the anus as well as the genitals, and the perineum. Lower limbs, they are located in the vicinity of the ankles, knees and feet.

Through self-care and meditation, Qigong can assist a person to achieve a calm mind. In a state of rebirth, or a new state of awareness, the person who practices of Qigong is able to experience the benefits of tranquility and peace as they experience the peace and clarity of their inner awareness. If you're wondering when is the best time to do Qigong It is important to know that the standard recommendation is to do it in the morning. It is the time when the Qi is at its best since there isn't any stress or tension and the level of pollution is lower. But, you're free to practice when you feel like, and you're not restricted in your practice of Qigong like you do you would in the morning. You have this same freedom throughout all of the time you practice. at first you'll find it more relaxing to do it for a couple of minutes. As you progress to an experienced practitioner, you'll be able to expand the length of your practice in line with your progress. It is generally accepted that Qigong is a practice that can last for a few minutes to an hour, with each person being able to choose the length of their practice. It is only necessary to practice at a time that you find suitable and the duration you feel at ease.

In the event of an illnesses, it is recommended to exercise Qigong regularly to help stimulate your body's natural healing processes in the body. The most experienced practitioners of Qigong consider that the practice stimulates the self-healing process by doing general or specific exercises to treat various health conditions.

A lot of people are eager to begin with their own experiences in Qigong. Qigong and are flooded with questions arising from natural curiosity. Most newbies are interested in the way the flow of Qi feels. In order to be able to answer these questions we must mention that every person feels the flow of Qi in a unique way. The most varied variations have been reported by Qigong practitioners. Some reported feeling the sensation of tingling, while others have reported the hands as swelling. A lot of people refer to the flow of qi as a heat sensation that engulfs them, or like the force of an invisible force were in control, but not their own.

But, the main issue to be addressed is how do I know in the event that I do not sense the movement of Qi? There are many people who are unhappy; because they don't experience the flowing of qi. they believe that they don't practice Qigong in the correct way. Actually, it's nothing to worry about if you're not experiencing the flow Qi. In addition, it is essential not to be concerned about these things, since you'll be unable to achieve the purpose to practice. The mind is in a state of tension and trying to figure out the reason and you'll be unsuccessful to achieve the state of relaxation. In certain situations that you are being unable to feel the flow of qi could be due to obstructions within the body, because of different injury, pain, or other misalignments. However these issues can be identified by an knowledgeable practitioner and addressed by routine practice Qigong.

It is important to be aware that there are a variety of fundamental postures that are recommended for practicing Qigong. The most common sitting positions require that you sit in the chair with your spine straight and your feet on the floor and your legs separated from each other. To achieve this position, you must to relax your muscles on your face and keep your mouth shut, and with an occasional smile. Another way to do this is that you sit in a cross-legged position with your spine straight and your hands resting on your laps. The half lotus posture can be used to assist in the practice of Qigong in which one must sit with the left leg beneath the left thigh, and the right foot underneath the knee of one's left. To do this hands are placed at the knees with ease. It is also possible to exercise Qigong from a supine position You must lie back on your back with your arms close to the body and your legs straight. The sideways-laying posture is an option to do Qigong exercises. You have to lay on your back with knees bent slightly and the other hand to provide support. The standing posture is widely employed to practice Qigong exercise, which requires standing with your feet spaced apart with your spine straight and your knees bent slightly. Not to be left out is the walking position, where the breathing is controlled by the slow movement.

Chapter 15: Historization Styles , And Effects.

The earliest traces of Qi Gong may extend as much as 2700 BC and Huang Ti, the legendary Yellow Emperor. The legend says that Huang Ti trained in Dao Yin, a form of exercise, which is translated as "guiding (or the) the energy'. The practice could have stemmed from shamanic rites from the past or the patterns of dance that are magical. Around the second century AD Hua Tuo developed the 'Movement of Five Animals' also known as 'Five Animals'. Ko Hung the alchemist had an 18-movement form and Da Mo or Bodhidharma as his name was initially known prior to arriving in China created a series of exercises that were taught to the Buddhist monks at the Shaolin Temple to build up their bodies so that they could stay in meditation for longer durations of time. These were later compiled as the renowned Tendon Changing and Marrow Cleansing Classics (Yi Chin Ching and Hsi Sui Ching).

As interest grew for Qi Gong in the 1980s during the 1980s, it was during the 80s that the Falun Gong movement emerged, proclaiming the synthesis that combines Buddhist as well as Taoist principles. The large number of people who practiced within the school (estimated to be 70 million at the time of the close in the 90s) caught the eye of authorities. Following peaceful protests against media bias, Falun Gong was banned by the Communist Party in 1999.

A variety of cultures across the centuries have believed in inner energy, also known as life force. It's even present in our modern version of the Star Wars, the epic myth of heroes'. There's a Japanese version is Ki while for Hindus it's Prana which is also known as it's the Serpent Power, Kundalini. The Qabalists also have Chiah.

Aristotle and Hippocrates believed in pneuma, which is also known as breath as being the essence of life. George Stahl, court physician to Frederick William 1 of Prussia thought of the anima being a vital force. In addition, Hans Driesch's Vitalist theory and the elan vital. Carl Reichenbach's theory of Odic force as well as Franz Anton Mesmer's "animal magnetism", Wilhelm Reich's Orgone Energy, the concepts that are part of Vril along with The Norse Aethm, and Native American Indian and Shamanic equivalents.

There are many types and styles that are part of Qi Gong. Certain styles are closely linked to Medical models like meridians, yin/yang

Polarity and those who believe in the Wu Xing or Five Element theory. There are also gentle stretching exercises which work joints and muscles. Some exercises could be prescribed for specific conditions as well as others that are designed to aid in the improvement of martial art abilities. Additionally, there are Buddhist as well as Confucian styles, as well as those of the Taoist ones.

Where Western exercise tends to exert stress upon the muscular and circulatory/respiratory systems, such as jogging, gymnasium work-outs, sports and aerobics, Qi Gong works on a subtle and seemingly indirect way of improving physical function by such means as adjusting structural alignment and taking into account the whole pattern of individual constitution, strengths, weaknesses and tendencies. Thus, there is a gradual improvement in overall health as the body adapts to new habits and there is also the advantage that exercises can be maintained into old age, as opposed to the more strenuous, popular types of exercise. Instead of engaging in muscular contraction the focus is on the relaxation of muscles and energy production, not the consumption of energy. It may sound odd however a sense of strength is not the goal for during Qi exercises, but rather it is a feeling throughout the body of effortless, loose power or the feeling of being connected.

The main impact that is a result of Qi Gong exercise is benefit to the lymphatic, cardiovascular and nervous systems as well as an increase in the strength of tendon and muscle. There is also evidence to suggest that it operates at a profundity level to improve the immune system as well as improve the health of bones and cells. could be uneven instead of a consistent progression due to the fact that internal blocks of energy are cleared. There may be the beginning of a worsening in some symptoms while the body adjusts to improve its functioning. It's as if the body is a consciousness. It can act at random or even send messages to us, such as when we consume food which isn't healthy for us. If the psychosomatic state of the familiar 'comfort zone' gets altered , there will be an adjustment period. the most important thing is to continue. The mind is everywhere in the body and is not restricted only to the brain. It is at least an alternative perspective, following several years in Cartesian duality.

The process of detoxification of Qi Gong could lead to unexpected emotions arising. In this instance, one must think of it as an energy pattern being released to help achieve a more balanced in well-being.

In reality Chinese medicine is based on the shocking idea (to an advanced Western perception) that the organs of the body possess their own unique form of consciousness (although this idea can be discovered in the earliest Greek philosophy).This is actually an analogy to help create an entirely new method of becoming conscious of the internal aspect of health that is often overlooked due to a focus on the physique of our bodies. When you awake in the morning, it is recommended not to get to get up too early since the heart could asleep. To take a quote from Jaynes yet again, 'Consciousness can have no physical location other than what we imagine it does' (op. cit., p.46).

After a time, the practitioner will become increasingly aware of "feeling of an inner balance. It's not a panacea. Each person has to assess their health or inability to maintain it as a whole image of their lifestyle and diet, the environment as well as relationships, work and routines. The blatant nonsense in a number of Chinese published publications on the subject might be due to mistranslation or due to an over-ambitious desire to be awed. Sometimes, the claims are interesting and relate to the realm of Chinese theatre, like masters shining light out of their hands. This is certainly a valuable skill for times I've returned from a night out at night with no moonlight and struggled to insert the door's key into the lock.

The basis the practice of Taoist Qi Gong can be easy to summarize; it involves standing, sitting and walking. Although there are some variations on these actions but it is considered that they are connected with the 3 powers (san cai) of Heaven, Mankind and Earth as well as the 3 precious treasures (san bao) of Essence, Spirit and Qi (there is a similar triune teaching within the Dzogchen lineage of Buddhism and the three treasures of Nature, Essence and energy). Heaven (Ch'ien) has Yang energies, Earth (K'un) is Yin (as in Mother Earth), and there is a balance between (Jen human). The essence of our Jing is stored in our kidneys and is connected to the experience of birth before birth as that is, the Waters of Life when we were suspended in amniotic fluid. Qi Gong and Tai Chi are believed to boost the kidney's energy, particularly kidneys acting as receptacles of energy that we have inherited. The postnatal energy we acquire which we are able to create is Qi. Shen is our spiritual energy, which penetrates our physical body; it is within us , and is also around us, similar to the concept that we have an aura.

We begin from the first moment of silence, commonly referred to as Wu Chi, or The Void as a meditative or empty state of possibility from where all our actions come from. It is imperative to be completely empty before we are able to fully experience any thing. A mind that is empty can allow us to detect the energy blockages in our bodies and respond with a sense of instinct in the fighting arts, as well as develop an awareness of the spiritual. This is then followed by Prenatal Energy, the spark of life, which is our primary inheritance. Postnatal Energy is the form of vitality that we gain and manage in our everyday activities, which includes our interaction to others as well as the

One way for you to fully experience the efficacy that is Qi Gong requires you to practice it in a way that balances the theory and the practice. Chinese students typically didn't doubt the lessons they were taught, they simply followed the instructions. The thought of thinking too much can block the Qi! If we're truly engaged in our activities, we lose our own thoughts and are able to engage in spontaneous actions and effortless activities, Wu Wei. The saying goes that 'Breathing is to be empty and waiting in the waiting for Tao'.

Al-Ghazzali The Persian philosopher in the 11th century said that theory is away from reality, that a state of travel to mystical perception is not comprehensible to the method of discourse used in science.

23

Qi Gong

24

Qi Gong

25

Qi Gong

26

Qi Gong

27

Qi Gong

28

4. THE HEALTH CLASSIC

The Neijing often referred to by the name of Yellow Emperor's Classic, is an amazing Taoist text that posits an integrated view of the concept health being linked to the surroundings. The message it proclaimed some four thousand years ago was a reality that the modern world is slowly realizing that we are completely separate from the natural world. The only reason we are coming to the same conclusion regarding the indivisibility of all things, and not the fragmented, piecemeal approach from the Aristotelian method The wisdom of these masters from the past being recognized.

The foundation of diagnosis is Wu Xing or Five Element Theory and the balance between Yin and Yang in line with Western medicine's notion of Homeostasis, which is the maintenance as well as regulation of the steady internal state. The many biological elements that are involved in this equilibrium process like respiration, and the maintenance of the major organ's core temperature are all accounted for according to the energetic model in which all systems are interconnected.

The exterior, back and upper portion of the body is categorized as Yang, while the inside is lower and front half are classified as Yin. The meridians, or channels of energy are connected to form Yin/Yang pairs. Liu the.

The lungs, the heart the liver, spleen and kidneys are Zhang and organs that are full or administrative which are related to those of the Five Elements; the Heart's element is Fire, Lungs Metal, Liver Wood Spleen Earth and Kidneys Water.

The Fu open or responsive Yang organs include the gall bladder, small and large intestines, bladder, stomach and the Triple Warmer or San Qiao (a concept of metabolism that serves a particular purpose of distributing energy from the primal across meridians of the kidney system in the development of prenatally). Triple Warmer refers to the three chou or levels of the body, the upper respiratory and circulatory system, the middle digestive, and the lower reproductive/eliminative functions.

The Pericardium is a different conceptual system that doesn't adhere with traditional Western Medical model. While the Triple Warmer transmits Qi and is connected with the lymphatic system as well as connective tissue, the Pericardium functions as an important transport channel to The Shen or spirit that lives within the heart.

There are two phases of Wu Xing. Wu Xing; generating and controlling. (Chen as well as Ko). The cycle of generating comprises of Water Metal, Earth, Fire and then back to water and the cycle continues (Water creates Wood that produces Fire, etc.). The sequence that controls the cycle are Water, Fire, Metal Wood, Metal, Earth, then back to Water and so on (Water is the one who controls Fire and Metal controls Fire.).

The seasons are regarded in the Wu Xing and have their affects on the body and so do the diverse emotions that are linked to the Zhang organs. One theory is that each organ are 'inhabited' by a dominant spirit. For instance, the Heart's Shen has mental, imaginative properties and the Lungs' Po conducts strength and endurance and the Liver's Hun has the ability to create ESP and The Spleen's Yi is rational, and the Kidney's Zhi regulates the survival drive and can also control.

The colour of the eyes is also linked to organs and is part of a visualisation method of sending healing energy to the affected areas.

The twelve meridians as well as their activity or Qi flow is linked to the seasons and each of the 365 points in the body correspond to calendar of the year's 365 days. It is evident that this kind of correlation is not difficult to dismiss from an allopathic perspective however, the idea is symbolic for the human body (microcosm) becoming one with the universe (macrocosm). In reference to the Hermetic rule: 'As above is what follows below'.

Prescriptive considerations consider the lifestyle, geography diet, and climate. A variety of variables for every individual situation would be assessed. The first step to diagnose is looking at the appearance of the patient and examining the pulses.

There may be imbalance or deficiency in the energy level of an organ. The balance of Yin and Yang applies. "Tonify the weak, calm excessive' can be a common principle, but it is a need for an exhaustive analysis of contributing factors.

The most important factor, according to Huang Ti, to effective healthcare is the balance of Yuan Qi. In the Yang Sheng Tao, the Way of Cultivating Life, established a healthcare system. This was the Western version was known as the Hippocratic Corpus of the Hippocratic Corpus, an assortment of medical writings that was likely written by other authors , as along with Hippocrates whose primary explanation of health was also built on an elemental model which was in this case the four Humours. The body fluids included blood, black and yellow Phlegm, bile and bile and their properties of cold, heat, damp and dryness matched Empedocles Four-Element Theory of the structure of the four elements that comprised all Matter (Fire, Earth, Air and Water).

Autopsies were not allowed in the Han dynasty, this could have affected the research of more intricate physiological processes as well as an inner contemplative method. The circulatory system was recognized and explained by the Nei Ching, which was written centuries before the discovery of William Harvey's the pulmonary circulation.

As Western religious sensibilities have shifted outward on the personifications and attributes that are God and Christ similarly, medicine has been able to see organic research as a fragmented and separated from the entire. The West the predominant view of treatments is specialization. Therefore, there are specialists in heart and eye specialists. They also specialize in every kind of disorders and illnesses. That's not to say this is not a successful method to treat. The director of the film John Huston, when asked what he believed he owes his long life to, simply replied"Surgery.". The Western allopathic medical method has saved the lives of many and can boast the benefits of X-rays as well as the finding of penicillin. However, there are areas where it may go off the rails.

This is the main distinction in Chinese medicine: the evaluation and treatment of the cause rather than symptoms. In Chinese medicine, symptoms are taken as indications of the body working to restore the balance. They don't view these signs as health threats to ignore, instead, but as something that needs to treat. Treatment of the individual and not the illness.

Another distinct feature is the concept of energy. In Western medical texts, the only reference to energy is within the area of psychology and the 'psychic energy. The case of China along with other Eastern nations, it has reached an extremely sophisticated level, with the co-relation of such concepts like the 8-part diagnosis technique (hot-cold internal-exterior, weak-weak and Yin-Yang) as well as the five Element Theory of Ko and Chen the meridian system, animus and p'o concepts and a myriad of other aspects.

Don't get caught up in the "Mystical Eastern". It's had its fair share of decades of war as well as poverty, oppression as well as class conflicts and ignorance, like the gruesome practice of foot-binding the Manchu Dynasty. China was at one point described as the 'sick person in Asia'. An understanding of psychological issues can be thought to be lacking.

Of course, any culture comes with its flaws in terms of political and ideological shortcomings. The Chinese civilization has made amazing advances in the fields of science and art. It is said that, for the Chinese it is it is it is believed that the Industrial Revolution is recent history. The statement is not intended to be interpreted as a negative way and is rather a way to highlight their vast past.

Reverting to the individual , rather that the universal, believe there is a reason to question the Western importance of external evaluation of the body.

The feeling of being well-being cannot be derived from an ideal state of being, just as being healthy isn't necessarily synonymous with being fit, or the reverse. The supposed norms of physical fitness are actually a fictitious notion. Typing people is absurd as can be seen when taking the time to look around the crowd. There is no standard case. We are all being typed (short and large and fat) to make it easier for the media due to the fashion and advertising industries and various corporate interests seek to establish an ideal physical appearance that is fiction. To live up the expectations of others is exhausting, and we don't do justice to the diversity of humankind and our many types of existence.

With that said it is important to be striving for our own personal feeling of perfection, but not to the degree of obsession or denial and not because it's normal to want to improve ourselves and live an ideal lifestyle.

29

Qi Gong

30

The Health Classic

31

Qi Gong

32

5. BREATHING

The Breath Is the God of Strength'. Chinese saying.

Breathing is a distinct physiological process that is able to be controlled by conscious thought and also an autonomous task.

The Physiology of RESPIRATION

The thoracic cavity comprises the ribs, the sternum and intercostal muscles, as well as the 12 thoracic vertebrae, as well as the diaphragm. The lungs fill the space and the heart is located between. The the apex of each lung sits slightly above the clavicle while the base is located on the diaphragm. The trachea is divided into two bronchi and then into alveoli, bronchioles, and capillaries. Each lung is protected by a membrane known as the pleura.

The rhythmic contraction of the diaphragm and the intercostal muscle is triggered by impulses from the respiratory center in the Medulla Oblongata. There are two main movements that occur during breathing: breath inhalation as well as exhalation. When the diaphragm contract, the chest cavity expands in the vertical direction, and also in a lateral direction from one side as well as from front to back due to contracting the muscles of intercostal. As you exhale, the relaxing of the muscles pushes air out. Carbon dioxide and oxygen are exchanged during the breathing process. Oxygen, which is absorbed by the mouth and nose, enters the lungs through the capillary and alveolar membrane. It is then absorbed by haemoglobin, a protein found in red blood cells and transported to the heart and later all over the body. CO_2 is an organic waste product, is exhaled.

Now, you are conscious of your breathing and what you feel when you breathe in and then exhale. Be aware of your breathing rate, whether it's either slow or fast irregular or regular deep or shallow. Be aware of any tension in any specific area of your body when you breathe. Feel your breath as it moves through and out of your body.

The method of breathing used through the mouth in Qi Gong is called Diaphragmatic or abdominal breathing. The diaphragm is thought to be the core of strength. It is believed that by focusing on the lower portion of the torso, breathing becomes more deep and stimulates the entire lung capacity. This technique can be used successfully by, for instance opera singers. The term is often used to describe it as filling the abdomen with breath' however, this isn't necessarily anatomically correct , but it does provide an impression of the method. Simply, when breath is inhaled, your abdomen expands, and when you breathe out, it contracts. For an example, during a Qi Gong exercise the attention is directed to the navel which is the center of power for Dan Tien. Dan Tien.

While in the majority of explanations for this technique, only the forward and reverse movement of the abdomen is thought to be however there is an spherical component, because the ribcage extends laterally the diaphragm raises and drops, and if you place your hands on the region that is between your kidneys or the Ming Men, as you breathe, you'll be able to feel a small motion there as well.

Exhalation is an Yang activity, as in the first moment of creative inspiration inhalation or the out breath, or "Word of God'. Exhaling refers to one of the stages in Yin withdrawal. The cosmological or religious speculations about the future of the universe may be formulated as the breathing cycle.

Pranayama is the yoga equivalent to Qi breath exercises includes numerous methods, such as closing your nostrils in a series of intervals while you breathe and counting to four on the in-breath, and 2 on the out-breath, etc. There's a possibility of anecdotal tale of a yoga practitioner who was so busy engaged in conscious control of breath that he lost his autonomic control, and then spent the night in a state of anxiety, trying to regain it. In either case, there's an important warning in the form of an Occam's razor. Applying this wisdom, the

North"If you're in doubt don't hesitate to act'. Alterations in breathing could alter the blood chemical composition and affect the cerebral function in addition to causing various other organic ailments.

The method known as Rebirthing was invented during the late 1980s, through Leonard Orr. It is described as "Conscious Connected Breathing," in which there is no gap between exhalation and breathing. It is believed that the body's "cellular memory' (memory that is dispersed throughout the body, not limited to cerebral) is activated by this process, and release previous traumas , such as birth issues. It has been accused of being simply over-breathing or hyperventilation which may cause panic attacks and tetany. Israel Regardie used hyperventilation as part of his job as a psychotherapist. in his book 'The Eye in the Triangle' he made the comparison between it and pranayama finding similarities between the two states of physical and emotional states (in this regard, he can be thought of as an earlier Rebirther).

Qi Gong tends towards minimum interference, or even making more efficient what is naturally. It is best to stay cautiously. While there may not be some benefits to exploring the different types of breath exercises, however, the most straightforward method appears to be the most effective and definitely safe.

The pathways to increase energy flow have to be created slowly. As with the development of an alignment of the body's structure Slow and steady exercise is essential to establish new connectivity.

The Embryonic Breathing technique is a very smooth and quiet breathing, that is, a piece that is made from tissue papers or feather is held before the nose, without being interrupted by the breath. You may notice it happens in a natural way and without any effort, when your concentration increases as you work out.

Another Taoist method I'll mention since it's been often mentioned in numerous books, particularly in relation to Taoist Alchemy It is also called Reversed (also known as Prenatal) Breathing. The abdomen is contracted when you inhale and expands upon exhaling. It can also be used in martial arts but it shouldn't be employed for prolonged durations. It is essentially a method to boost the energy.

When Taoist teachers speak of breath that is 'whole they're speaking of the movement that occurs throughout the body when breathing for example, how knees relax and straighten while exhaling and inhaling while practicing in standing Qi Gong.

When it comes to combining movement and breath, for instance, in the "active" Qi Gong exercises, then typically the breath, in the form of Yin breath will be connected to an upward or downward movement, while The out Yang breath, however is generally a downward or falling movement. For instance, the opening in an Yang form Tai Chi form consists of arms being elevated towards your body to ensure that the wrists remain an approximate level with the shoulders. This is when you breathe in. As the arms lower, you exhale. It is also an Qi Gong practice in itself also called Taoist Water Exercise. Taoist Water Exercise.

The breathing rate during Qi exercises should be approximately similar to that for Tai Chi form, around two breaths out and in per minute. However, you should adhere to the pace that is comfortable for you. Be careful not to force the breath.

Breathing is the constant interaction with the world around us, as we continuously take the elements all around us, and then emitting the energy we converted. The lungs are never idle. There is a belief that through breathing one can also create changes to the environment. Personal alchemy.

The main goal of Qi Gong is to use breath to increase the health condition and overall well-being, in addition to spiritual considerations.

33

Qi Gong

34

Breathing

35

Qi Gong

36

6. SITTING

"The best way to be will Be' (Lao Tzu).

There are many positions and formal postures that are suitable for sitting meditation, including Seiza or "correct sitting" to be found in Japan ('sitting meditation is Zazen).Taoist sitting meditation is different from the typical posture of seated Eastern meditations in that it does not emphasize the half-lotus or lotus posture and feet's soles are set flat on the floor. Similar to kneeling and sitting on the ground, sitting isn't always comfortable in Western societies, and there is a study in which it was found that there are physiological distinctions between cultures more comfortable with sitting on the ground than we are, for example the knee joint being more robust. These positions do not assist in the flow of energy externally and internally which is the basis of Taoist practices.

The chair-seated posture demonstrates the general principles of Qi Gong physical alignment of not being overly relaxed, to the extent that you're likely to sleep and not allowing tension in the body through striving to do too much.

It is believed that the Qi Gong posture in a chair is the middle between these extremes. It is at ease, but still straight. The legs of the upper limbs should be horizontal and in line with the ground. The lower and back legs should be vertical. This posture is often referred to in the form of the Lightning Flash, as it is similar to the zig-zag pattern that is representing lightning bolts. It is also often referred to as The God or King posture, which is based on the sitting Egyptian statues of Pharaohs. The hands are put on the knees with hands up.

It also creates a clear pathway between Heaven energy flowing from the top of the head as well as the palms, as well as Earth energy coming through the soles of your feet that are connected to the ground. It is ideal for the 'neutral spine' the natural 3 curvatures of the healthy spine: which include the cervical, thoracic, and lumbar. The ideal posture is to maximize the function of circulation and breathing.

The benefit of this situation is that it is able to be utilized for a purpose that is beneficial anytime you're in the mood or are able to remember it. You can use it on a bus or train, or even at work. Simply taking a few deep breaths can aid in calming your mind.

In the next step, you will encounter sitting meditation sitting on the ground at the conclusion in the Yuan Qi set of exercises You will notice that this pose involves putting the soles of feet together in order to create the energy loop. The goal of Taoist sitting meditation is principally to control. We are constantly distracted and depleted of energy by our senses being distracted due to noise pollution and calls on our attention and the depleting effect of our digital environment. Most people cannot allow themselves to be in a space of their own thoughts and instead require the safety of being connected to headsets, mobile phones, and TV screens to keep them from the outside world and from themselves. When we can stop the 'Monkey mind that is a constant tangle by thoughts of the past or future, we're simply being present. According to Jane Roberts in 'The Nature of Personal Reality' stated it: "The purpose of power lies being present in the present moment'.

Concerning the psychoanalytic method The psychoanalytic approach isn't the best way to analyze the contents of the unconscious, which can be described as simply processing your stuff. That is the source of the suffering of Sisyphus. It is better to follow the perspective to the creative. The power of visualization is a powerful tool and the power of creative visualization can be used to direct or guide energy.

Meditations that are guided that imagine scenes that are joyful events or locations that one's life has or even imagined places, can be peace. At first, I tell that people to be calm and to let them observe their thoughts as they drift around their minds. an initial step involves to keep the body stilland taking deep breaths without fumbling. This is a major challenge for some. Fear of silence is the same as an fear of darkness. Additionally, refraining from talking is an exercise in and of itself. The constant talk can drain vitality; avoiding conversation is believed to protect the meridian Qi. The practice of sitting quietly is known as Jing-zuo.

It is the Inner Viewing practice of Nei-shih or the Nei-kuan method involves imagining the inside of the body. It is a prelude to other exercises like the 'Inner smile', where organs are smiling at (yes I know that it sounds crazy but the idea is not without logic: the positive energies). It is also synchronized with the use of various coloured energy that is believed to permeate every organ, based on The Five Element theory. Since different kinds of energy states are attributed to each organ , there is a psychological alchemical component that transforms negative thoughts and emotions. Taoist mantras and chants possess additional health-enhancing and altering characteristics. They clear the mind of the normal state by using an unfamiliar language, encourage the feeling of tuning in' to the present or ancient tradition, in the field of acoustics suggests, they are a vibrational influence on the body.

Subvocal vibrations of sound is a possibility if you are lacking privacy, however it is less effective. "The six healing sounds (Liu Zi Jue) is a well-known Qi Gong using the intoning of various sounds to resonate with internal organs (liver heart, spleen, liver kidneys, lungs, and livers and the Triple Warmer) or, to be more specific by harmonizing with the PRF, or Prime Resonant Frequency of every organ. This is not an uncommon idea considering the effectiveness of ultrasound therapies as a standard treatment.

Ni Hua Ching is a teacher. Ni Hua Ching has provided numerous fascinating invocations, like Yi Shi Vi which he is akin in the manner of the Three Tan Tien, and he employs words of Chuang Tzu or Chuang Tzu in addition to other.

What you can learn from sitting quietly regardless of whether you invoke invocations and/or not is a feeling of your inner state, which is derived from the feeling of the bones, muscles, and organs that make up the body's physical structure. Making use of mantras to aid in Taoist practice isn't the same thing as using "Affirmations" or "Positive Thinking'. These aren't effective (see p.105 of "The Path of Least Refusal, The Powerlessness of Positive Thinking" to see a definitive response). Positive thinking differs from imposing positive thoughts, which might not be in harmony with your perception of reality.

In order to make a brief reference to what's known as 'Inner Connections These are the gods that are thought to be a part of the body and the Universe. The process that involves merging an image with a person,, known as "Assuming a Godform" in Western rituals of magic is known as 'Visualizing the Valley Spirit' in Taoism. Lao-tzu is the most sought-after choice to accomplish this.

To get the body moving to the next stage, which could be a moving or standing I often add Mo meridian points massage towards the end of the meditation session. The next three points are lung Meridian Points. LU1 as well as LU2 are situated just below the the collar bone, just before the shoulder bulge. The LU5 region is located on the elbow's crease beyond the Biceps Tendon.

Points are usually found as small depressions (perhaps this is the reason they are referred to as cavities) and might be tender when pressure is applied. Massage with both fingers by rotating them pressing into the point, but not forcing.

Furthermore, Ren 17 on the midline between the sternum and halfway between the nipples, has the potential for opening as well as a an energizing effect.

What we've begun to discover by simply sitting is that mental concepts can be amplified by intention and how the body can be receptive to suggestions. It is important to note that we engage in sitting as an active process. Sitting for long periods in a straight posture could create stress in the back and, of course, many medical studies have found that a lifestyle of sedentary living could increase the risk of developing conditions such like heart disease and diabetes. The ideal posture for sitting for a long period of period of time, according to medical advice is to lean back 45 degrees with your back supported naturally.

37

Qi Gong

38

Sitting

39

Qi Gong

40

7. STANDING

"Patience is a virtue of the highest order'. Chaucer.

The first exercise that we do is standing. It may seem odd however there is an enormous amount of work involved in learning to sit still. It involves a thorough understanding of your own anatomical alignment, respiration awareness, our individual state of stress or relaxation as well as balance and concentration. In reality, you will find that there's plenty of movement in a state of stillness, particularly on an internal level. When practicing Qi Gong the mind is more active when you are standing position than sitting or lying down.

The physiological benefit of being upright is that it's more comfortable to hold our big heads upright, which allows for more space for vision and moving weight vertically. This is combined with our hands that are nimble (freed from the necessity of walking with four limbs as other mammals do) to provide us with an efficient way to make use of our muscles. 40 percent of our body weight is composed of skeletal muscles. The downside is that the joints in the lower part of the knees, hips, and ankles are now required to bear the weight of our bodies by transmitting force to the floor.

The place you stand is the center point of your existence and the Omphalos ('navel'''), originally a stone object used to signify a central location like the Temple of the Delphic Oracle). Towers, trees, ladders and mountains all signify the same relationship between heaven and earth (hence why Mt. Fuji as in Japan in Japan and Kun-Lun in China as sacred mountains that represent their countries). In its aspect of being the symbol that is"the" Tree of Life the human body is an axis that runs through the entire world. "Standing like the Tree is a well-known description of exercises that require standing.

In the beginning, the empty stomach, or even an excessively full one could affect your mental state Therefore, it is recommended to have small snacks at least one hour prior to exercise, and wait one hour after exercise before having a meal again.

ENVIRONMENT AND TIME

Sunrise is the optimal timing, or at least early in the morning, for energetic workouts, since you're ready for the rest of the day. It is best to practice outside but it's contingent on the weather and season. Doing Qi Gong sitting on the ground or grass without shoes in natural settings like a park, near a lake, or among trees, is recommended. You shouldn't be too hot or cold. Images as well as stories about people who practice in the desert or snow are typically of masochistic martial artists, and it's got to be mentioned. There is no need to be adversity (too too much) to master this art even though standing in a single position for long periods of time demands an amount of determination. Certain teachers even specify the direction to face; South ideally. This instruction could be affected by circumstances like not seeing the sun directly in your eyes.

The wind is believed to disperse Qi So, you should be aware of that even if you're working inside and there's a breeze. It is essential to have a peaceful environment. It is away from people and pollution and noise, as much as possible. It is important not being distracted so this is also a good reason to disconnect or turn off your mobile, and making time to yourself.

CLOTHING

No tight belts, no restriction. An uniform isn't required, but some instructors find wearing something similar to that Tai Chi style outfit helps to enhance the effect, and puts practitioners in the correct mindset. I wouldn't suggest Chinese style slippers , which have slippery soles of the plastic. Simple canvas shoes such as Espadrilles can be worn. It is recommended to take off watches and jewelry, since they can cause interference.

STANDING POST (ZHAN ZHUANG)

The stance that is the basis of it is called Wu Chi. Wu Chi stance, Wu Chi being the name used for the state of absolute the infinitude of nothingness, or emptiness.

In the beginning, it may be beneficial to stand before a full-length mirror to examine your posture. Begin by standing with your feet the same width. Imagine you're walking on parallel lines and that the outer edges of the big toe as well as the heel of each foot are upon the lines. Check your balance.

Then, shift your weight slightly onto your heels. A little over the middle in the sole your foot, you will find Kidney 1, or K1 which is a meridian-point. K1 is sometimes referred to as Yong Quan (Bubbling Wells or Bubbling Spring) Point likely because of the earth energy that flows through it. There are a few Qi Gong instructors suggest curling the toes to elevate the sole slightly however, I find it generally creates tension that is difficult to sustain initially Therefore, it is best to relax the feet.

Breathe in deeply and exhale, then slowly lower your weight back, as if you're getting ready to sit on the chair.The knees shouldn't be bent forward to the toes. A mirror will assist you in determining the correct position until you're accustomed to your posture.

The coccyx points down and the spine is straight. Chuang Tzu said, 'Take your spine as your principle of regulation'. If you take a look at an anatomical representation that shows the spinal column, you will see that it isn't completely straight, however, it has four curves: those of cervical, thoracic pelvic and lumbar, each curving back and forward. However, it's more convenient in this case to imagine the back as straight. Place your chin down slightly and notice the upward pull upon your back as you do it. To take inspiration an idea from Alexander Technique, imagine a golden thread hanging from at the very top of your skull (the Bai Hui or Du Twenty Point) from where your body hangs.

Relax your shoulders. The neck and shoulders are two of the regions of the body where we may be carrying loads of tension since we tend to be more upper-body concentrated.

Relax or'sink' your chest. It is recommended to adopt the opposite effect of the'soldier on parade ground' posture in this regard, that is, don't enlarge the chest.

The arms should hang to the side. The inner edges of your hands including the space between the thumb and forefinger at the point referred to in the field of Hegu or LI4 rest on the thighs , so that the palms are facing in the opposite direction. When the arms are in this position, the elbows are angled to the side, allowing room at the axilla (armpit) both sides.

You can either look straight ahead or down to an angle (still making sure your head is straight) or if you are distracted by visuals then close your eyes.

You feel as if you are sinking into the earth. Your knees shouldn't be carrying weight, they are joints for weight transfer. In the spirit of standing like a Tree' imagine that there are roots growing from your feet, similar to those of trees down to the ground. This is even true if you are in a room and not on a level floor because it's an exercise of imagination however, it can affect your sense of balance as well as "groundedness". Find yourself below your body and above your head.

If you do not have a breathing problem, your mouth should be shut so that you can breathe into and out of your nose. The tongue's tip is connected to the mouth's roof and not too far away; it should be between the front teeth on the upper side.

After having inspected all of the points of alignment The following step is ease into it. There is an Chinese word "Sung," which is translated to something that resembles relaxed awareness. It is being alert and not inactive. This is the state we want to achieve when the body gets settled into the posture. The body will adapt itself, and we don't want to strain to get outcomes. It's possible to have to deal with the old patterns of your posture, and you may experience discomfort and aches at first. The pains are normal and go away with continued training. A specific pain can be warning signs. If you feel pain immediately stop the exercise and evaluate the severity of the issue.

It is advised to keep the posture simple initially. There are a variety of different types in Standing Post that involve holding arms in various positions, however as they tend to create tension, they should be kept until later, after the person has had experience in sitting in a definite position for a long period of time. Also, putting the arms straight can hinder the fundamental components of the posture.

While standing, you'll notice your legs starting to shake. Even if you are strong in your leg muscles because we're not utilizing muscular strength during the exercise , but for form integration. Keep breathing and relax. The shaking stops after a few minutes or be replaced by a gentle and pleasant "buzzing" sensation. If shaking continues to occur then stop the practice. It is not advisable to push yourself too hard in the exercise, but it's not the case of "no pain, no gain'. Similar to Tai Chi, once you have your legs in order then everything else will follow.

Try the step-by-step approach to relax each portion of your body, from the top of your head down to the toes. Notice the difference when tighten the muscles of your forehead, by frowning. You will feel the tension all the way all the way until the peak of your head. Release the frown together with a out breath. Then work your way down the the body this way by extending your fingers to the arms downwards through the trunk, and then down the legs until your toes. You can also imagine your focus as a transverse line of light slowly moving down from the top of the head down to the feet, melting away any tension.

As you progress, gradually increase the length of time you have. Every person is different in how much time is beneficial. Even a few minutes to relax is beneficial. Begin by increasing the time to an hour, and then work up to. On the other end of the spectrum are martial artists who utilize a standing posts as the main power training method used in The Chinese internal style of martial arts and who are able to maintain an erect stance for up to an hour or more. There's a point at which there are decreasing returns at this point. If you stand for an extended duration of time during an exercise, tension can creep into the body and you'll be aware of things such as shoulders that have almost invisiblely lifted. Release tension by dropping it to the ground by exhaling. When standing, release is always downwards, towards the ground.

When you are in the more advanced, higher arm positions, more stress will be felt on the shoulders and the lung points on in front, between the chest and shoulders may be tense. Additionally, the upper back and neck. If you feel that heat is rising towards the head, take a deep breath or blow it out with your mouth several times to eliminate the sensation. You should immediately end the session if you feel that it is still happening.

After a while , you realize that the most difficult obstacle to solve is your personal mind. In the classic texts like the Dhammapada explain to the mind, it is the adversary. It has to be eliminated! The beast is definitely tamed.

There are excuses that pop out of not practicing and distractions, boredom. Be aware of your thoughts floating through the air like clouds, and let them to drift away. Keep committed. One way for you to get positive results is to be consistent.

Music is useful as background music, specifically to aid in keeping track of time since you don't want to constantly keep track of your clock. If you know the length the piece is, you won't be focused on what time it is and how long you've held the stance , and how long you've held it. The use of heavy metals at full blast isn't advised.

Conclusion

The many different Qigong systems are the result of many different generations of practitioners, who've spent years working to improve their techniques and theories to attain their goals.

There are simple techniques as well as others that are very vast and complicated. Most of them are based upon medical theories and must be understood in order to reach the highest level.

It typically requires the supervision of a certified instructor and a certain amount of training based on the system being utilized. It's really hard and probably impossible to impart this knowledge via books. It is definitely not possible if you wish to only learn through books.

It is equally real that it isn't essential to know the entirety of a qigong technique or be a renowned practitioner to gain its advantages.

The goal for this text is to examine in a basic and straightforward manner the practices that are used in the majority of Qigong methods and the benefits they bring to us.

I particularly rely on the instruction that my teachers have taught me on the way I train in. A Treasure to health"In it, I offer an overview of the various types of Qigong. I discuss the background of Luohan gong, its goals and the methods used to achieve them. I also outline the most important elements of its application.

The strategies I present in the book inspired by that method.

To realize that our body, energy and mind. To realize the ability to function with breathing, movement and concentration. It is important to realize that they are three distinct elements that must be integrated. Learning simple exercises that will aid in improving them could be a great starting point to increase our well-being.